FEAR NO EVIL

Fear No Evil

Facing the final test of faith

David Watson

Foreword by
James I Packer

HODDER AND STOUGHTON
LONDON SYDNEY AUCKLAND

Copyright © 1984 by Anne Watson

First published in 1984 by Hodder and Stoughton,
a division of Hodder Headline PLC

This edition 1994

The right of David Watson to be identified as the author of
the Work has been asserted by him in accordance with the
Copyright, Designs and Patents Act 1988.

10 9 8 7 6 5 4 3 2 1

British Library Cataloguing in Publication Data

Watson, David, 1933–1984
1984 Fear no evil.—(Hodder Christian paperbacks)
1. Cancer—Religious aspects—Christianity
I. Title
248.8′6   BT732

ISBN 0 340 59807 7

Printed and bound in Great Britain by
Cox & Wyman Ltd, Reading, Berkshire

Hodder and Stoughton Ltd
A Division of Hodder Headline PLC
47 Bedford Square
London WC1B 3DP

Acknowledgements

When Edward England, my literary agent and personal friend, suggested that I should attempt a book of such an intimate and painful nature, I was unsure. Increasingly, however, I felt that it is important today to talk openly about cancer, especially from the standpoint of the Christian faith. Edward's advice, and that of Ann, his wife, has been marvellous throughout. I am so grateful.

Hilary Saunders, my indefatigable secretary, has not only typed several drafts of the manuscript admirably, but has constantly encouraged me, gently corrected some of my writing and throughout has helped us all as a family during the most difficult year of our life. My gratitude to her is profound.

Other readers have helped considerably: Carolyn Armitage of Hodder and Stoughton, John and Gay Perry of Lee Abbey, the Very Reverend David Edwards, Provost of Southwark Cathedral, and Teddy and Margaret Saunders whose personal support, together with many others (especially in London and York) has been of the utmost value.

Especially I thank my Team: Mark and Carol Slomka, Sandy Campbell, Alison Charles, Margot Evans, Shaun Islip, Mark Jennings and Diana Nairne. Not only have Mark and Carol made many perceptive comments about the manuscript, but the whole Team's constant prayer and love has been quite extraordinary.

The debt I owe to many other friends is almost endless. Most of all I thank God for showing me his love as never before.

To John Wimber, Blaine Cook, John McClure,
Bishop Morris and Anne Maddocks,
together with countless Christians throughout
Great Britain and overseas who have prayed, loved
and encouraged us as a family.

Contents

Foreword

When David Watson, evangelist, author, and renewal preacher, died of cancer at the age of 50, a great man fell in Israel, as the thousands who poured into his two memorial services in York and London attested. But David's ministry is not over; though dead, he still speaks by his books, and not least by this, his final piece of writing. *Fear No Evil* is, quite simply, marvellous: poignant and radiant, matter-of-fact and sublime, modest and heroic, heart-rending and heart-warming in equal measure, and all the more overwhelming for being understated in David's very British way. To introduce it, as I have been asked to do, is the privilege of a lifetime. In doing so I want to pinpoint what seems to me to be its real greatness.

'Our people die well,' said John Wesley (a leader, incidentally, with whom David bears comparison in a remarkable way). Wesley was celebrating God's grace among the Methodists. Until recently a good death was seen as the godly man's crowning achievement, the climax of his good life. That is why tracts on the 'art' of dying were among the first printed books in all European languages; that is why William Perkins, the Puritan devotional writer (with whom also David bears comparison, though whereas Wesley died at 88, Perkins died at 44), composed *A Salve for a Sicke Man (The Right Way of Dying Well);* and that is why from the sixteenth to the nineteenth centuries, when most adults died in the presence of family and friends, great importance was attached to a Christian's deathbed sayings. Things are, of course, different today: death has replaced sex as the great unmentionable. All stress among Christians is laid on present knowledge and enjoyment of God, and the old awareness that only one who is ready to die can live to God's praise has been generally forgotten. The discipline of what Alexander Whyte called 'forefancying your deathbed' is in abeyance, and anyone who were to hint that he wanted his death to edify others would be thought unbalanced for thinking about his death at all. But we are the unbalanced ones, and there is something here that we need to relearn.

Readers of *Pilgrim's Progress* will recall the unforgettable last scene in which the pilgrims crossed the river of death to the Celestial City. Mr Stand-fast, the last to go, experienced 'a great Calm in the River': 'when he was about half-way in, he stood a while and talked to his Companions,' and this is what he said.

'This River has been a Terror to many, yea the thoughts of it also have often frighted me. But now methinks I stand easy . . . The Waters indeed are to the Palate bitter, and to the Stomach cold, yet the thoughts of what I am going to, and of the Conduct that waits for me on the other side, doth lie as a glowing Coal at my Heart.

'I see myself now at the end of my Journey, my toilsome Days are ended. I am going now to see that Head that was Crowned with Thorns, and that Face that was spit upon, for me.

'I have formerly lived by Hear-say, and Faith, but now I go where I shall live by sight, and shall be with him, in whose Company I delight myself.

'I have loved to hear my Lord spoken of . . . His Voice to me has been most sweet . . . His Word I did use to gather for my Food, and for Antidotes against my Faintings. He has held me . . .'

While Mr Stand-fast was saying this, Bunyan tells us, he was taken. 'But Glorious it was, to see how the open Region was filled with Horses and Chariots, with Trumpeters and Pipers, with Singers and Players on stringed Instruments, to welcome the Pilgrims as they went up, and followed one another in at the beautiful Gate of the City.'

To any Bible lover with a full-grown Christian imagination, Bunyan's pictures in these paragraphs and those that
surround them trigger joy and tears, ardour, adoration, and
assurance, with a power that no other Christian literature
can match – though some things in Charles Williams and
C S Lewis, all modelled (I think) on Bunyan, come close.
But few of us in this century know our Bibles very well, nor
have we full-grown Christian imaginations, and Bunyan's
diction may strike us as merely quaint. Must we then miss
the ministry that his lyrical prose has had to so many in the
past? Not necessarily. For God in grace has given us our
own Mr Stand-fast, who paused during his own dying to
model for us in contemporary terms faith face-to-face with
the last enemy. That was David's final role, and his blow-
by-blow record of a losing battle with cancer is his equiva-
lent of Mr Stand-fast's last speech. The same certainty of
God's love is voiced; the same victory of faith shines forth.
That is the greatness of *Fear No Evil*.

The fact that David, right to his last page, hopes for
supernatural healing that never comes is not important. In
the providence of God, who does not always show his
servants the true point of the books he stirs them to write,
the theme of *Fear No Evil* is the conquest of death – not by
looking away from it, nor by being shielded from it, but by
facing it squarely and going down into it knowing that for a
believer it is the vestibule of glory.

David's theology led him to believe, right to the end, that
God wanted to heal his body. Mine leads me rather to say
that God evidently wanted David home, and healed his
whole person by taking him to glory in the way that he will
one day heal us all. Health and life, I would say, in the full
and final sense of those words, are not what we die *out of*,
but what we die *into*. Whichever notions fit, David's or
mine (and differences will continue about that), there is
profound wisdom in David's maxim that the *what*-question
(what, Lord, are you saying to me, doing for me, asking
from me?) gets one further than the *why*-question (why,

Lord, has this happened?). To ask God to give us an account of himself and his actions is a dead-end street, as Job found, for God doesn't do it. However, to know God in Christ – that is, to know that God is Jesuslike – is to know that he is always ready to tell us how he loves us and how we are to love him, even when he will tell us nothing more about his present plans. But to know this, as David knew it, is to be unsinkable – whatever the enemy, the battle, and the wounds. David lived and modelled this even more tellingly than he verbalised it: read this book, and you will see.

Samson, we are told, did more for God by his death than he had ever done in his life. In character terms, one could hardly imagine a person less like Samson, the lifelong juvenile delinquent as he has been called, than the tidy, disciplined, courteous, poised, genial, and humble Cambridge man that was David. Yet he may well be like Samson in this one regard. Could it be that his dying testament will minister more widely, helping more needy people, and at a deeper level, than anything he wrote before? Could it be that God has accomplished more for his kingdom by taking David home as he did than he would have done by any alternative pattern of events in David's life? Most certainly it could. I know no book better fitted to impart to twentieth-century Christians in the West the lost wisdom about death than this one. I am more thankful for it than I can say. I must not keep you from it any longer.

James I Packer

Introduction

All of us, I think, have deep-seated fears about something in our life, even if they are seldom expressed. We may be afraid of all sorts of things: spiders, mice, moths, snakes, injections, loneliness, exams, feathers, failure, the dark, the dentist, flying – the list is endless. Most are frightened of death. And of all the terminal diseases that may afflict us, none causes such anxiety as *cancer*.

When I first heard earlier this year (January 5th, 1983 to be precise) that I had cancer, the news hit me like a thunderbolt. All human hopes and securities were suddenly shattered. 'It *can't* be true,' I said to myself foolishly and anxiously. 'That sort of thing doesn't happen to me!' But it did, and my deepest fears were realised.

Often I say, as a Christian, that I am not afraid of death but I am sometimes afraid of the process of dying. In my mind I think of several people I've known who have died painfully and rather horribly from cancer. My fears have not been groundless.

With the fear of cancer so widespread in society, I was encouraged to write this book, giving an honest account of my feelings and reactions and how I have come to terms with cancer over these last eleven months. I write unashamedly as a Christian, although I hope that my thoughts will be of some interest whatever faith a reader may have.

One test of any religion is how far it will stand up to the crises of life, especially the final crisis of death. The shock of having to come to terms with death made me examine again the whole basis of my Christian faith.

I have tried to mingle my personal story with my own

wider reflections, because such thoughts have all been with
me since the diagnosis was made. The experiences of this
year, although mild compared with the pains and traumas
endured by others, have made me ask searching questions
about life and death. I have been candid about my doubts
and fears, even though I struggled through to a restful trust
in God and in his healing power. Even now, eleven months
later, I am quite vulnerable to further fears, especially in the
middle of the night.

It has not been an easy book to write, partly because I am
still standing too close to these events. At the same time I
record my thoughts as someone who is right in the middle of
the trial, with no certain security about the future – apart
from faith in God and in his healing power.

The problem of suffering is always a baffling one, devoid of
simple solutions, and yet the experience of that suffering is all
around us. The question is, how can we live with it, face it,
overcome it, and reach that position where we *fear no evil*?

1

Anxious Moments

'Have you got any spare room in your cupboard for a chest of drawers?' I asked Fiona. 'And Anne, where on earth can we put these two chairs?'

'Hang them in the garage, with everything else!' replied Anne. The garage was already looking like a warehouse for old second-hand furniture, with chairs, tables, old carpets and mirrors hanging on its walls.

'There's just *not* enough room!' complained Guy, as he heaved his bed into another corner of his room.

It wasn't really as bad as all that, and in fact we are extremely fortunate to be in such a pleasant house in central London. But it was the first time we had ever moved as a family. For seventeen years Anne (my wife) and I had lived in York, and since Fiona was sixteen and Guy thirteen, it was the only home they had known. I am an Anglican clergyman and we lived in a large and typical mid-Victorian rectory – not very attractive, but it had fourteen main rooms and a considerable garden which usually looked wild since we had little time to spend on it. However, it was *home*.

Suddenly, all our roots had been pulled up, as though all our teeth had been pulled out in one go. It really hurt! We moved from north to south ('They've got such funny accents!' said Fiona and Guy), from one of the most beautiful small cities in Great Britain to the heart of a huge metropolis, and from a rambling house that had been almost a part of our lives to a small house in a mews. Even though we gave away masses of tables, beds, wardrobes, desks, chairs, carpets and clothes, we still carried far too much with us, and it was quite a game squeezing it all in. Anne and I saw it mostly as the next adventure in our lives. Fiona and Guy longed to be 'back home', in York.

Sam missed the big house and garden as much as anyone else. Sam was our dog – a friendly mixture of every breed you could think of, though appropriately fierce with intruders. But Sam wasn't well. The difference between York and London hit us hard when Sam had an operation two months after our arrival. Virtually the identical operation had cost us twenty pounds in York; in London we paid one hundred and thirty-four pounds – considerably more than my week's salary! And a few weeks later Sam died. Anne sobbed, the children were upset, and I really missed him too.

The move to London had not been easy in all sorts of ways, and I found it hard to answer Fiona's constant question, 'Why did we leave York?' Basically we had moved because of my work, and because Anne and I believed that God had called us to London, but it wasn't easy convincing our children, who were missing 'home'.

Then came the biggest shock of all.

I had gone to my doctor, William Robarts, for only another prescription concerning my asthma. Since I had learned to live with asthma for eighteen years it was no more than a brief routine visit.

'One little question,' I asked him as I got up to leave, 'Does this medication have any side-effects? I seem to be going to the loo rather a lot these days.'

'How long has this been going on for?' He startled me by the serious tone of his question.

'Well I'm not sure. I haven't paid much attention to it until the last few weeks. But looking back I suppose it might have got gradually worse over this last year. As you know I travel widely, and any problems I've put down to changes of food and water. I remember having a little trouble in Sweden nine months ago . . .'

'Do you mind if I have a look?'

After a slightly uncomfortable examination he looked thoughtfully at me across his desk. 'You have an ulcer in the colon. I would like you to see a specialist because you might need an operation. It could be serious.'

'I'm afraid that is impossible,' I replied, beginning to feel uneasy. 'I'm just off to California with my team for five weeks, and of all the events in the year this is one that I simply cannot cancel. It's out of the question.'

I spend much of my time travelling to many parts of the world with a team of about eight men and women who are gifted in the performing arts: music, song, dance, drama and mime. In five days' time we were due to leave for our most demanding tour of the year: five intensive but enjoyable weeks based at Fuller Theological Seminary in Pasadena, California, with weekend engagements at San Francisco, Phoenix Arizona, Fort Leavenworth Kansas, and one or two other places. I was already booked to lecture over sixty times (including a few preaching commitments) and I knew that over eighty pastors were coming from all over America and from as far away as Australia for those lectures. I teach in California at the same time every year, and I always find it totally exhausting but wonderfully stimulating. It stretches my capacities to the full, yet I always come back with a renewed vision of God and of his work in different parts of the world. No, that was one engagement I definitely could not cancel! My doctor, however, seemed unmoved by my protests.

'Are you saying it could be – malignant?' I asked, a little nervously.

'It's possible.'

I did not know what to say. My heart thumped away beneath my outward poise.

'I'll just make a phone call,' said my doctor; and within a couple of minutes the appointment with Mr Beard, a consultant, was fixed for the day after next.

'This really *is* serious,' I thought to myself, almost as

though I was dreaming, expecting to wake up at any moment to discover it was only the start to a nightmare. But no, I was wide awake. It was no dream.

As I stepped out of the doctor's surgery I could not really believe that anything was seriously wrong. It is true that I was shaken, but I could not accept the possibility of an operation. I wove my way through the January sales' shoppers streaming in and out of Peter Jones department store. It was late afternoon, and the lighted streets were thronged with brightly coloured punks from King's Road and fashionably dressed ladies from Belgravia.

Sloane Square seemed alive with colour and bustle, shopping bags bulging with bargains and bright lights from Christmas decorations still shining from the trees. I always love the start of a new year. From earliest childhood I have thought of it as a season of promise and hope – a new start and fresh expectations. It is Epiphany, the manifestation of Christ to the world when the wise men from the East brought their priceless gifts to honour the infant King. Every year seems to herald the dawn of a new age.

I felt sure that my doctor was only being cautious. I felt remarkably fit. How could I have a malignant ulcer? Indeed, what exactly *was* a malignant ulcer? I noticed that neither my doctor nor I had used that dreaded word 'cancer'. As I looked into the faces of the shoppers hurrying home for tea I wondered how many of them carried in their hearts secret fears, anxieties and sorrows? I walked through the quiet elegance of Eaton Square into the jostling crowds around Victoria Station. I was going to buy a brief-case with some money that had been promised me for that purpose. And it would be a brief-case for California. I really could not cancel that trip. I was almost certain that I would be going with my team on the Tuesday as planned. The talk of a malignant ulcer was surely no more than a sobering scare. In fact, purchasing the brief-case for the journey became for me a symbol of faith. Or was it of fear? I found just the one I wanted and I hurried home.

'How did you get on at the doctor's?' asked Anne once I had displayed my brief-case.

'All right. He thinks I may have an ulcer,' I replied cautiously.

When our children, Fiona and Guy, went out of the kitchen to watch television, I closed the door and related to Anne what had happened.

'What actually did he say?' pressed Anne. She had been trained as a nurse at Guy's Hospital and would not be satisfied with anything less than the full details.

'He thinks it could be malignant,' I replied, speaking in short sentences since I wasn't far away from tears. 'Got to see a specialist. Mr Randolph Beard. Friday morning, nine o'clock.'

I sat there, choking back my emotions and watching her face. Anne had been through some rough times in our marriage, and a few lines on her face and the wisps of grey hair spoke of pain and tears. But she was still beautiful, with open searching eyes.

'Mr Beard is the best!' she said enthusiastically. 'He was loved and respected even when I was a nurse.'

'I'm glad,' I replied weakly.

We held each other's hands and prayed.

'Heavenly Father, we know you love us and are fully in control of our lives. Help us to trust you, and keep us in your peace. We really need your help. Amen.'

Anne cried a little. We gave each other a hug, and then I went to join the children in case they wondered what was going on.

'What did the doctor say?' asked Guy immediately.

'Just that I've probably got an ulcer, and may need an operation,' I replied as casually as possible.

'An operation? Gosh!' Guy was puzzled, since the only ulcers he had known were in his mouth and had not needed an operation. But I didn't try to explain.

We spent the rest of the evening watching a film on television. It wasn't a good one and I couldn't concentrate, but at least I was with my family and I relaxed.

That night I took a mild sleeping tablet, committed my life, my family and my future to God, and slept well.

The next morning I met with the team as usual, mainly for a time of worship and prayer. I began by telling them the news of my visit to the doctor, the possibility of an operation, and the uncertainty of my going to America. They were all shaken by the news. For weeks we had been preparing for this trip, but essentially the team were going to illustrate *my* lectures. Apart from packing, we were all set. Now, at the last moment, everything looked precarious.

Much more important, I knew they were very worried about me. Although the members of the team were all half our age Anne and I had come to love them dearly as our Christian brothers and sisters, and we were not surprised by their immediate and enormous concern. We joined together in several songs of gentle praise, expressing our faith in God's ultimate control and unceasing love; and then we prayed for one another. They gathered round me and laid hands upon me, praying that God's peace would continue to fill my life. I felt immensely encouraged, and returned home, leaving the team to rehearse for California, but without much enthusiasm.

Back in my study, I tried to work further on my lectures. I had not written the material for two of my subjects and others needed tidying up. But my mind was not in it! My natural apprehension unsettled my stomach more than ever, and I seemed to spend much of the day in the smallest room in the house! Some work, however, was accomplished. In the afternoon I made good progress on the two lectures whilst spending an unusually long time in the dentist's waiting-room – a wonderful place for gathering one's thoughts!

That evening I was restless and anxious. There was still plenty to do in preparation for California, but the possibility of my going seemed to diminish hour by hour, and I really wanted to spend more time with Anne, Fiona and Guy. So we had a quiet evening together doing nothing in particular.

Friday, January 7th was a bright and fresh January morning. The air was crisp and the winter sunshine seemed full of hope. I went to see the consultant, Mr Randolph Beard. Arriving early, I walked through the streets until my appointment was due. I was surprisingly peaceful as I rang the doorbell and was ushered upstairs to meet Mr Beard. At once he impressed me with his quiet and encouraging manner; I could see why Anne had enthused about his outstanding reputation as a consultant-surgeon.

After a brief examination he spoke gently. 'You're in real trouble. You have a malignant ulcer and you need an operation at once.'

I was stunned. My worst fears were confirmed. I felt my throat getting dry with tension. Feebly I told him how difficult an operation was at that time, with over sixty lectures to give in California in a few days, and with many pastors coming having already spent hundreds of dollars on this course. How could I possibly cancel the engagement at this stage? Mr Beard smiled kindly, but was unbending in his decision.

'I cannot overstress how important this is,' he said.

I had no choice but to accept his guidance. He told me that, in anticipation of my visit, he had provisionally reserved a bed for me in Guy's Hospital and that I should be there first thing on Monday morning. He warned me that almost certainly I would need to have a colostomy (I had only the vaguest idea of what this meant), but that many active people learn to live with one. He made it clear also that I must be off all work until Easter at least, with no international work for six months.

As I left his surgery my head was spinning. I still could not quite believe that this was happening to me. I was worried about Anne and the children. How would they take it, I wondered? And what about my trip to America? How on earth could I sort that one out? What about all the pastors coming at considerable expense to themselves? And what about all my other numerous engagements? How could I disappoint so many thousands of people? We had been planning Christian festivals in various towns for months. Everything seemingly depended on my remaining fit and well.

What on earth did the future hold? Indeed was it 'on earth' at all?

2

Roots

I remember little about my father. He was away in the Army for long periods of time, and died in India in 1943 when I was ten.

My earliest memories go back to the North-West Frontier of India, now Pakistan, where my father was commanding a mountain-battery of guns. I have childhood impressions of gunfire over our bungalow, topis and polo-ponies, Indian servants and beautiful saris, and even finding a hooded cobra in my bath! We came back to this country in 1937, when I was four. I must have been a romantic child for I proposed to a five-year-old girl on Victoria station having just crossed the ocean seas with her. To my dismay she refused me, and it took me another twenty-seven years before I summoned up the courage again – but it was not to the same girl!

My father's death was particularly tragic since he was a Christian Scientist and, according to his beliefs, refused all medical help when he was seriously ill with broncho-pneumonia. My mother, stunned by the effects of such convictions (which she never shared) had me baptised and confirmed in the nearest Anglican church, although I understood absolutely nothing of what was going on.[1]

This confusing religious start to my life, coupled with the dull monotony of formal school chapel, caused me to explore a variety of religious paths. Having rejected Christian Science, I dabbled in spiritualism to see if I could make

[1] I have written my story more fully in my autobiography *You Are My God*, Hodder & Stoughton, 1983.

contact with my father. My uncle, however, was a devotee of
Rudolph Steiner, and I went on to study the Law of Karma.
This led to forms of Buddhism and to belief in reincarnation,
which for me at the time was the only logical solution to the
problem of suffering. For those afflicted in this life, there was
always the promise of a better reincarnation another time.
Not that there is any scrap of real evidence for this, of course.
It was purely one interesting theory. I also tried several more
obscure religious philosophies as well.

Becoming increasingly disillusioned, however, and react-
ing strongly against the hypocrisy (as I saw it) of Army
religion during my two years of National Service, I turned
my back on God and became an atheist or humanist. I went
up to St John's College, Cambridge, with mathematics and
science as my subjects, but switched instead to philosophy,
psychology, logic, ethics and metaphysics. This was effectively the humanist faculty in the university. We felt that
the only hope for mankind was for us to work out our own
destiny in the best way we understood with our rational
minds.

During my first week at Cambridge I sampled all the
societies, whether I believed in them or not, primarily to get a
feel of university life. I was amused to find myself at a
tea-party organised by the Christian Union, but I was
impressed by the speaker, a clergyman called John Collins. It
was not so much *what* he said but the *way* in which he said it
that struck me. He seemed obviously genuine as though he
was speaking from a first-hand experience of God.

I talked to him briefly afterwards, and the next day we had
breakfast together whilst he explained very simply, step by
step, how I could find God in my life. What he said made
sense, although I knew he could not prove it. I also knew that
I could not prove my atheism. He spoke warmly about the
reality of God found through a personal relationship with
Christ. I realised logically that it might be true and equally
that it might not be true. If it were not true, forget it; but if it
were true, it was quite simply the most important truth in the

universe. The honest thing to do was to conduct an experiment in the realm of faith.

That night, having read a helpful booklet covering much the same ground as that which John Collins had explained to me, I knelt down by my bed and asked Christ, if such a person really existed, to come into my life. I meant what I said, although I was disappointed that I felt exactly the same immediately afterwards. Later I came to see how that simple unemotional step of faith became the most important turning-point in the whole of my life, eventually affecting every area of my being as I deepened my knowledge of God.

Certainly I needed help, which was wonderfully given in my first year by David Sheppard, who had recently been the Captain of England's cricket team and is now the Bishop of Liverpool. I had to think through carefully my new-found faith, for much of my academic studies challenged every basic Christian belief. It was a testing time, and I waded through plenty of doubts before I gained a better intellectual grasp of the integrity of the Christian faith. During my university days I found such joy in leading some of my friends to Christ and seeing them built up in the faith, that it was hard to do justice to my philosophical studies (although I did tolerably well in the exams).

It was not long before I believed that God was calling me to the ministry of the Church of England; and after two years training at Ridley Hall in Cambridge I was ordained in Rochester Cathedral and joined John Collins at St Mark's Church, Gillingham in Kent. I had three marvellous years in that predominantly dockyard parish, and saw the power of Christ changing the lives of people who had come from a very different background to that of Cambridge.

After three years, however, I went back to Cambridge, this time to the Round Church where I was gradually drawn into further work amongst students. That period in Cambridge was marked by three major personal events. First, I was one day consciously filled with the Spirit of God and felt the love of God enveloping my whole being – I fell in love with Christ.

Secondly, and nearly a year later, I fell in love with a beautiful girl who is now my wife. And thirdly, a short time before our wedding, I developed severe asthma which has been with me, on and off, ever since.

Partly because of the asthma, but there were other reasons as well, the first few years in our marriage were particularly stormy, and we both have a lot of sympathy for those with broken marriages. But for the grace of God ours would have been exactly the same. However, we worked through those storms to a much more mature and open relationship, and I think we have become more whole people as a result.

Then on Friday, January 7th 1983 I learned that I had cancer.

3

Quick Change

The weekend was a whirlwind of telephoning, rearranging, discussing and praying. High on my priorities was the question of how I could salvage my lecture tour in California, with so many clergy and ministers coming for an intensive course for which they had been studying and preparing. My team was ready to go since we had prepared ourselves carefully for our most challenging commitment so far; but we urgently needed one or two experienced Christian teachers whose understanding and approach would be almost identical to my own. Knowing the pressures on my own diary it seemed inconceivable that anyone with the necessary qualifications and experience would be available at this last moment.

Added to that, I was profoundly disappointed about not going there myself. This was to have been my fourth visit but my first time with our new team, and the first extended teaching period of a month (the previous periods had been only two weeks). There were visits arranged to San Francisco, Phoenix Arizona, the Grand Canyon and Kansas, not to mention the growing number of friends I knew out there. I really wanted to go. And now some instant re-thinking had to take place.

There is no doubt that I was worried about this as I made my way home from the consultant's surgery, although I prayed as I walked and believed that God knew all about the problems I faced and had his own solution for me. I am naturally impatient and I like to be in control of situations.

Through my Christian life I have always found it difficult to obey the instruction in the Bible to 'be still before the Lord, and wait patiently for him' (Psalm 37:7). If I do not have the immediate answer to a problem, I like to work it out myself as soon as I can. Some of my close friends tell me that I need to learn how to be still, how to listen to God, how to trust him when there are no apparent solutions, and how to wait for his guidance. As a born activist I confess that I find all this difficult, and yet I appreciate the wisdom of it.

On this occasion I did not have to wait long for an answer to my urgent prayer. By the end of that Friday morning, almost miraculously, I had found two outstanding replacements for those five weeks in North America. They were two friends of mine, David Prior and David MacInnes, both extremely gifted communicators and much in demand for their teaching and preaching skills.

'David,' I said to each of them on the phone, 'can you help me? It's rather an emergency. You see, I've got cancer and can't go to Fuller. Can you take my place?'

Both Davids were dumbfounded by my news and request. I could tell that they were shocked about the cancer and were trying their utmost to respond positively to the cry for help.

It was unbelievable that they could both be free and willing to accept such a massive teaching assignment at this eleventh hour, and equally remarkable that their wives were prepared to let them go. But it happened, and an enormous worry rolled off my back.

Later that day Fiona photo-copied all my lecture notes, Hilary, my secretary, sent them off to the two Davids, and I rewrote the closing paragraphs of my autobiography *You Are My God*. The manuscript was almost finished, and I sensed the urgency for completing it before going into hospital on the Monday, otherwise it might not be concluded for months. 'I heard only yesterday and unexpectedly,' I wrote, 'that I have to go into hospital in two days' time for a major abdominal operation . . . This has come as a total surprise, but I know that the matter is both serious and urgent.

Suddenly everything in the future has become uncertain, even life itself . . .' I still was avoiding the word *cancer*.

That word is still a highly emotive one in our modern society, and for most people it is inseparably linked with fear and death. It is sometimes called 'the Big C' or 'that dreaded disease'. There are no real answers at present to cancer. The word is almost synonymous with helplessness and hopelessness.

Later that day I rang a number of praying Christian friends to ask for their support. They were all stunned by the news. In particular I phoned through to a special friend of mine, John Wimber, the pastor of an outstanding church in Yorba Linda, California, where their healing ministry is one of the most impressive I have seen anywhere in the world.

John is a large, lovable, warm and gentle person, reminding me of a favourite teddy-bear. He also has an able mind, wide Christian experience and shrewd spiritual discernment. Every now and then in my travels I meet someone whom I feel I can really trust – someone who loves me and accepts me as I am, who is not trying to use or manipulate me, and who is full of godly wisdom. There are not many like this, but John Wimber is one.

His secretary answered the phone and explained that John was away on a staff retreat for the weekend and could not under any circumstances be disturbed.

'The thing is,' I said with the word sticking in my throat, 'I've got cancer, and I need help.'

'John will call you right back,' she replied gently and reassuringly.

And John did.

He listened as I told him the facts.

'David,' he said, 'the first thing I want you to know is that we love you. Secondly, I don't accept this cancer and I believe that God wants to heal you. Thirdly, I'm going to call the whole congregation immediately to urgent prayer.'

Both his words and his tone of voice were so encouraging that I just cried.

'Thanks John. I love you all too.'

That weekend John called his 3,000-strong congregation
to commit themselves in prayer and fasting for my healing.

On the Saturday morning I was joined by Teddy Saunders, Vicar of St Michael's, Chester Square and Chairman of
the Belfrey Trust (which finances and guides our work), and
Douglas Greenfield our team Administrator who researches
and plans all our festivals. Teddy, Douglas and I went
through the diary in detail, looking at the many engagements
fixed for the next eighteen months – most of which required
complex planning – to see which ones we had to cancel
outright, which ones could be 'put on ice', and which ones
could go forward with some rearrangements. In the following
six months alone we were booked for a mission in Wands-
worth Γ[.] on, and festivals of various lengths in Brighton
and Hove, Plymouth, Exeter, Bristol, Harlow, Norfolk, Bedford, Oldham and Folkestone. As well as that there was a
Lent series of seven lunch-hour services at St Lawrence
Jewry, in the City of London, and many other preaching
engagements. How could I cancel all those? Or what alternative plans could possibly be made at this stage? I am not a
brave person and am naturally frightened of pain; yet at that
moment I was far less concerned about my own future than
about letting so many people down. At the same time I was
increasingly sad about not being able to lead those missions
and festivals which I had been looking forward to for months.

I hated the thought of having to rearrange all those events.
For years I have loved this work. It has been a vital part of my
life. Suddenly to be stripped of it all was personally very
painful. I also felt as deeply committed to my team as they
were to me, and the thought of not being with them for at
least six months was distressing, and I was concerned that
they might be out of work because of me. My heart sank
continually as the implications of my illness hit me.

However, Douglas had come from an evening in Guildford
with the marvellous news that a good friend of mine, Bob
Roxburgh who had recently become the Pastor of Millmead

Baptist Church in Guildford, was almost sure that he could make himself available for several months to take festivals in my place together with the team. This was another great burden off my shoulders since I knew that the plans were well advanced for major festivals at Harlow and Bedford at least. I could feel the tensions within my body relax as the diary was cleared and as I realised that the vast majority of people involved would not be let down.

Anne and I found it difficult to know what to say to our children. With cancer being such an emotive word, we decided to leave it for the time being as 'an operation for an ulcer', and only fill in further details as they became necessary. I was amazed at the calm way in which they seemed to take it, although of course they were anxious – and no doubt picked up our tensions as well.

Throughout this time, Teddy and Margaret Saunders, who lived just round the corner from us, were marvellous, and so was Hilary, their daughter and my secretary. Our respective families had been on holiday together in the summer and, as family friends, we planned a relaxed afternoon to relieve the tensions of the last few days. We had a delightful lunch in their home, and then piled into our cars to go to Leicester Square, where a *Pink Panther* film was being shown.

It was a grey Saturday afternoon, and driving through the London streets seemed once again like a dream. 'I *still* can't believe it's all happening to me' was the constant thought going through my mind.

At the Odeon, Leicester Square some young man recognised me. 'Aren't you David Watson? How are you?'

How do you answer a throw-away question like that? 'Well actually, I've got cancer. How are you?'

Inevitably I made the usual polite comments and sat down to enjoy the film. Every now and then my mind turned back to the fact of cancer, and I was afraid. But on the whole I forgot everything with the hilarious actions and accents of Peter Sellers. Laughter is one of God's great gifts and a delightful means of relaxation. Life is not always very funny, and my own situation was far from humorous, but laughter can save us from the deadly snares of self-pity and self-importance. It can also act as a powerful antidote to disease by turning negatives into positives. As we emerged from our two hours of happy escapism I felt better equipped to face the major battles still to come.

4

Getting Ready

There had never been a Sunday like it.

As usual I woke early, washed and dressed, and spent some time reading my Bible and praying. After breakfast we went as a family to a Communion Service at St Michael's Chester Square.

Ever since I was twenty-one I have put my trust firmly in Christ, convinced that he was and is the Son of God and therefore the supreme authority in matters of faith. The substantial evidence for this has always seemed totally compelling. When it comes to the most critical issues that ever face us, I would rather trust Christ than any other person in the history of the world. And we all have to trust someone, because nobody knows what happens at death. Who else, apart from Christ and his resurrection (the evidence for this being overwhelmingly powerful) can give us any solid hope for the future? There is no one. Yet one day we must all die, and then what? We remain agnostic in the face of death only by ignoring the many promises and warnings given to us by Christ. Everyone, without exception, has faith in one direction or another: either faith in Christ, with all the weighty evidence for that, or faith in supposing that what Christ said is not true or not important. Sadly, it is often only when our faith faces the final test that we begin to consider these questions seriously.

Brendan Behan, the Irish poet, once confessed, 'I'm a daylight atheist.' It is easy to say 'there is no God' when there is no immediate challenge for personal atheistic views. But the atheist has faith – he cannot *prove* there is no God. In fact the atheist has far greater and more daring faith than the Christian, since he must hold to his non-belief against all the teaching of Jesus Christ. Moreover, Christ not only taught with astonishing authority about the vital issues that affect us all – life and death, God and man – he also vindicated the truth of what he taught by the matchless character of his own person. The Christian has faith, yes, but his faith rests firmly on the historical facts of Christ and his teaching. The atheist has to believe that all those things are not true – where is the evidence for that?

For many years I had been telling people that I am not afraid to die. I know the reality of Christ in my own experience. He has made God real in my life, and has promised that one day he will welcome me into his home in heaven. At the same time, with the sudden and alarming discovery of cancer, I realised that the time had now come to place the whole of my life into God's hands once again and to renew my trust in him for all that lay ahead of me.

That simple Anglican Communion Service in St Michael's said it all. When all the false promise of the world is stripped away like old wallpaper (or at least threatened), the only solid reality that matters before God is that Christ has died for us to bear all our sin, and has been raised from the dead, giving us a living hope in the face of our last enemy.

There were not many in the church that morning, perhaps sixty. But here was all that I needed as I faced a future that was suddenly insecure and uncertain.

> God so loved the world that he gave his
> only Son, that whoever believes in him
> should not perish but have eternal life.

Quietly I confessed my sins to God, thanked Jesus for dying for me, and told him that my life – and the future of my family – was in his hands.

> Christ has died:
> Christ is risen:
> Christ will come again.

I took the bread and the wine, tokens of Christ's ultimate
sacrifice for my sins and the guarantee of God's unchanging
love and mercy. I knew that I belonged to him for ever. Not
even death could separate me from his love.

> Through him (Christ) we offer you our souls and bodies
> to be a living sacrifice.

'Lord, I'm yours. You can do with me whatever is your
perfect will.' In that surrender I found his profound peace. I
was ready.

After lunch, a number of Christian leaders had been
invited to the home of Teddy and Margaret Saunders to pray
for me. We knew it could be a prolonged time of prayer, so
Anne felt it best to take Fiona and Guy out for the afternoon,
to avoid any undue anxiety on their part. Fiona rode on
Wimbledon Common, and Anne and Guy went for a walk at
the same time.

I was amazed that such extremely busy Christians could
make time on a Sunday afternoon to spend time with me. I
looked around the spacious drawing-room at mostly very
familiar faces, men and women whom I had loved and
trusted for many years. I knew they were all 'full of faith and
of the Holy Spirit' (a description given to some New Testament Christians), and we had an immensely encouraging
time of worship and prayer, during which they anointed me
with oil in the name of the Lord. This was simply following
the New Testament instructions: 'Is any among you sick? Let
him call for the elders of the church, and let them pray over
him, anointing him with oil in the name of the Lord; and the
prayer of faith will save the sick man, and the Lord will raise
him up' (James 5:14f). Often I had done this for others, but
now it was my turn to be at the receiving end of this loving

and caring ministry. Although the purpose of this gathering was serious it was a relaxed and peaceful time, and we still knew how to laugh!

Since these were all mature and experienced Christians I listened carefully to what they had to share with me. One said that she had been woken at 3 a.m. with a clear impression (which she took to be from God): 'This experience will not diminish David's ministry, but will in fact increase it.' I puzzled over this, since it seemed that exactly the opposite would happen, if not end my ministry altogether. However, others shared various verses in the Bible that had come to them as they had been praying for me: 'What I am doing you do not know now, but afterward you will understand' (John 13:7); 'You are my servant . . . in whom I will be glorified' (Isaiah 49:3); 'I will remove disaster from you' (Zephaniah 3:18). All those present seemed fully convinced that God was not only fully in control, but that he would glorify his name even more through what was going to happen and would add a further dimension to my work. I could not see how this could happen, and I experienced an inward struggle between *faith* ('Lord, I believe this and thank you for it') and *fear* ('They're only trying to encourage me, and anyway God could be glorified through my death!'). However it was not so much their words that helped me but their obvious love and concern. They really cared.

That evening I rang my elderly mother. Over the years since my own conversion at twenty-one, she had come into a living faith in God – a faith that was often surprisingly strong in difficult circumstances.

'Hallo,' I said, 'it's David.' I knew my mother was surprised to hear from me on a Sunday.

'Is everything all right?'

'Well, I've got to go into hospital – tomorrow in fact – for an operation.'

'You haven't! Is it serious?'

'I'm not sure. It could be.' I went on to explain, as gently as I could, the events of the last few days. Although my mother, aged eighty-two, was obviously shaken by it all, she seemed full of faith, believing in God's power to look after me.

'I'm sure you will be all right. God will take care of you, and I shall be remembering you constantly in my prayers.'

It was not an easy phone call. I kept simply to the basic facts, but I was glad that she took it so well.

That evening I packed a few basic requirements for hospital, including my *Good News Bible*, which I knew would be the source of enormous comfort and strength in the coming days.

It could not have been an easy time for my family either. Guy was due to return to his boarding school the next day, so he was a bit tense anyway. Anne was packing for him, and trying to support me at the same time. Fiona was endeavouring to encourage us all!

We prayed, and went to bed.

5

Into Hospital

After breakfast on Monday morning I left for Guy's Hospital. It was hard saying goodbye to the children. Fiona, who like me is naturally rather fearful about hospitals, was outwardly calm but inwardly anxious. Guy was going off to school later that day, and so we would not see each other again for several weeks. Anne was marvellous in her support for us all, however, and Teddy Saunders drove us in his car, he and Margaret having postponed their sabbatical leave to South Africa until our immediate crisis was over.

'Well, there's no turning back now,' I thought to myself. 'The adventure has now begun!' I was much in prayer to God, and constantly aware of his presence with me as we entered the hospital.

I was immediately impressed by the pleasantness and quiet efficiency of the Sister in charge of the ward, and her manner set the tone for all the nursing staff there. Their cheerfulness and professionalism gave enormous encouragement to any nervous patient like me! I had been in hospital only once before for an operation (that was about thirty-five years ago) and all my life I have been ridiculously squeamish about such things as tubes sticking in or out of people's bodies. Because of this, hospital visiting has always been something of an ordeal for me throughout my ordained ministry, and only genuine compassion for those who are sick has helped me to overcome my fears.

Anne was on her old home ground at Guy's, and was wonderful in getting me settled into a little side room just off the main ward. When she was sure I was all right, she returned home to take Guy to school, but came back to the hospital later that evening and again first thing the next morning. I was now off all food since the biopsy was booked for the Tuesday afternoon.

The days of both the biopsy and the operation are little more than a blur to me now, although a number of features stood out. In the first place, contrary to my usual expectations, I was struck by the efficiency of the Church of England! The hospital chaplain came round twice, giving Anne and me Holy Communion on the second occasion and once more anointing me with oil in the name of the Lord – *not*, for the uninitiated, to be confused with the Last Rites! And my first visitors outside my family and close friends were the Bishop of Fulham coming on behalf of the Bishop of London, and the Bishop of Kensington. The two Bishops missed each other by half an hour, and I marvelled at being the object of such episcopal concern. I found both their visits encouraging; and letters, telegrams, cards and flowers began to pour in, assuring me of the prayers of God's people from countless different places. It was all quite extraordinary, but terribly moving. Most of the flowers had to be taken back to our home because their beautiful and powerful fragrance gave me a touch of hay fever. Anne replaced some of them with such realistic silk flowers that someone kindly watered them for me!

Most treasured of all were the letters from Fiona and Guy, which I read over and over again. They were mainly chatty letters, but Fiona wrote almost every day, which was amazing! I thanked God for them both and for the love of all my family.

The biopsy confirmed that the ulcer in the colon was malignant. I had already resigned myself to this fact, so it did not come as a shock. But the implications of the cancer had to be thought through, especially the ominous warnings about a colostomy. (In my layman's terms, a colostomy involves the sealing of the normal passage of the bowels, with an artificial opening being made instead in the side of the abdomen, to

which is attached a plastic bag.) I tried to imagine myself at
home and in public lavatories trying to deal with a colostomy
bag. How would I cope with this in the homes of other
people? The whole idea was repulsive to me in spite of
reassurances of how well people adjusted to this. Anne and I
had helpful instructions about the nature of a colostomy, and
how the bags should be used; and mentally I tried to prepare
myself for this structural alteration in my anatomy. The
cancer was so low in the colon that it seemed certain that I
would have a colostomy, and a bag was even attached to me
before going down to theatre, to give me some idea as to its
feel and position. I cannot say that I relished the thought of it
all, but I had a remarkable sense of God's peace as I faced the
unknown.

As I lay in bed I thought of all that had happened during
those seventeen years in York, the happiest period in our life.
When we arrived in 1965 we moved into a large but filthy
rectory, needing urgent redecoration in all its fourteen
rooms, with no money available for the purpose. My own
salary was £600 a year! The church, St Cuthbert's, had a tiny
congregation and was soon to be closed – probably to be
made into a museum. I thought of all the struggles as we
worked and prayed that God would bring new life into that
church: the time of Anne's deep depression and the time
when I nearly died from asthma.

And yet the work grew! I thought of those amazing
Thursdays when roughly 140 people would come into our
home, filling six rooms, for the purpose of Bible study and
prayer. This was the heart-beat of the new life that was
steadily developing. I remembered more than sixty university missions, which I had the privilege of leading, although
my continued absence from home was not easy for Anne.

My mind moved on to that extraordinary further growth
in the church when we moved to St Michael-le-Belfrey
(another church about to be closed and three times the size of
St Cuthbert's), when we held regular services in York Minster with packed-out congregations, when we lived in an

extended household, when we developed music, drama and dance groups and learnt how to express and communicate our faith through the arts. Above all, I thought of the incredible sense of love that blossomed in the congregation and the wonderful quality of worship. Although people came from all over the world to see what was going on, they were usually struck most by the love and worship.

It was far from perfect, of course. We made numerous mistakes and learnt a lot about forgiveness. But the church was alive and real. God was in that place. As I lay in my hospital bed, I knew that hundreds in York would be praying continuously for us as a family, and I thanked God for the incredible love and support they had constantly given us over the years.

When on my own, I spent as much time as possible reading the Bible, especially the Psalms, mingling prayer and praise. Psalm 16 has for a long time been a favourite of mine. I preached from it for my farewell sermon at York, and I have always loved a song based on this psalm:

> For you are my God;
> You alone are my joy.
> Defend me, O Lord.

The translation in the *Good News Bible* is particularly helpful:

> You, Lord, are all I have,
> and you give me all I need;
> my future is in your hands . . .
> I am always aware of the Lord's presence;
> he is near, and nothing can shake me.
> And so I am thankful and glad,
> and I feel completely secure,
> because you protect me from the power of death,
> and the one you love you will not
> abandon to the world of the dead.

You will show me the path that leads to life;
    your presence fills me with joy
    and brings me pleasure for ever.

Quietly, as I leant back on my pillow, I meditated on those words and let them sink deep down inside me.

'*You, Lord, are all I have.*' I knew that when death comes we have to leave behind everything and everyone. So as an act of the will I handed everything over to the Lord – something I have done almost every day from that time on: my work, my future plans, Anne, Fiona and Guy, other friends and members of my family, my health, my life, my all. One by one I released them to God until I could say in my heart: 'You, Lord, are all I have.' I had already found such riches in Christ that I knew that I would be more than content with that. No one else could offer me complete forgiveness. No one else could be with me day and night throughout my life, and even through the valley of the shadow of death. No one else could give me a new heart and a new life. No one else could give me an abundant hope in the face of death. There is no one like Jesus! If we try to hold on to the temporal pleasures we enjoy now, we may lose everything. But if, in our hearts, we lose everything to the Lord, we have nothing more to lose – in fact we gain our life, said Jesus.

'*You give me all I need.*' At this moment I was experiencing a deep and untroubled peace, on the brink of the biggest trial in my life. If Jesus could meet my very real needs now, I could trust him with everything. I knew that he would never fail me. I sometimes worry about possible future problems which seem far too big for me to handle should they ever arise. In the Bible we are promised that we shall find 'grace to help in time of need'. God's grace, meaning the resources of his love, is there when the need is there, but not in anticipation of that need. I surprised myself by the unusual degree of calm I experienced when even life itself was threatened. This is God's grace *in time of need*.

'*My future is in your hands.*' This was especially reassuring at a time when my future was completely unknown and perhaps distinctly limited here on earth. Often I had taught people, in Festivals of Praise, to give what the psalmist called 'the festal shout'.[1] God's people have always been encouraged to shout acclamations of faith, to encourage one another in the Lord. One festal shout I have taught many thousands of people all over the world is 'The Lord Reigns!' I have seen the faith and confidence of people rise up visibly by acclaiming the truth that God has the whole world in his hands. He is the sovereign Lord. He is ultimately in control. We cannot trust him too much. Now I could rest in the certainty that *my* future was in his hands, whatever the outcome of the operation might be.

In this way I went through the whole of Psalm 16, letting every expression take firm root in both my mind and heart.

'*I am always aware of the Lord's presence.*' To be truthful, I cannot always *feel* his presence – indeed I seldom feel it. But I am always *aware* of it, mostly because of his repeated promise that he would always be with me, but also by many years of proving that in my own life.

'*He is near.*' I 'practised' his presence with me, right by my bed, day and night, until I knew that nothing could shake me. I could honestly echo the words of the psalmist, 'I feel completely secure.'

As I spent time chewing over the endless assurances and promises to be found in the Bible, so my faith in the living God grew stronger and held me safe in his hands. God's word to us, especially his word spoken by his Spirit through the Bible, is the very ingredient that feeds our faith. If we feed our souls regularly on God's word, several times each day, we should become robust spiritually just as we feed on ordinary food several times each day, and become robust physically. Nothing is more important than hearing and obeying the word of God.

[1] Psalms 89: 15, RSV.

'*Your presence fills me with joy.*' My spirit was almost buoyant as I prepared for the operation. I knew that God was with me, right beside me, and I felt ready to tackle this new adventure with him. Quietly I rested in the assurance of his presence as I was wheeled down the corridor towards the operating theatre.

6

Death Sentence

My first conscious memory after the operation was feeling for the colostomy bag. To my amazement and immediate relief it was not there! Mr Beard had avoided a colostomy after all, though he later admitted that they had 'sweated' a little over it during the three-hour operation. I was profoundly grateful.

The next day, when I was a little more aware of what was going on, Mr Beard came with his retinue of medical staff. He explained how they had cut out the malignant section of the colon and had managed to staple me together with a Chinese staple-gun! My mind boggled at the thought of it. But, he went on to say, they had discovered that the cancer had spread a little into my liver. He looked at me straight in the eyes and said gently, 'This is inoperable, I'm afraid. And I'm very, very sorry.'

I smiled weakly, but it felt as though I had received a death sentence. Cushioned perhaps by post-operative drugs, I felt no great panic – just a helpless sinking feeling.

'How long have I got?' I asked.

'We can't really say. Perhaps a year. Maybe more, maybe less. I'm asking Dr Harper, a specialist in these things, to come and see you when you are a little stronger.'

I am not sure when the news made its full impact on me. I was totally unprepared for it and frankly stunned by it. I felt numb. Anne, who was sitting in the corridor at the time waiting to visit me, was shattered when she was told. It was a difficult moment for us all, and no one knew quite what to

say. It was one of those times when we were silently trying to
absorb the information that had shattered us so completely.
We were in a state of shock.

'Oh well,' Anne and I said to each other, smiling rather
weakly, 'we must learn to live one day at a time, and to thank
God for each day as it comes.'

My immediate reaction was to think that I had roughly
365 days more, so that the next day it was only 364, then 363,
and so on. This proved to be both depressing and crippling in
its negative effect. I had always imagined that for those under
sentence of death, the worst experience was probably not the
sentence itself but the agonising period of waiting. Every
morning you wake up with the same nightmare that does not
fade with the day since it is reality. Every night the same
dreams haunt you. Imagination loves to feed on fear, and the
result can be almost paralysing. Undoubtedly it can hasten
the advance of the disease and the moment of death.

Nothing Anne and I could think of encouraged our hope
for the future, as far as this life was concerned, although
thankfully we knew that our lives were in God's hands and
that not even death could separate us from his love.

But death would certainly separate us from one another.
When Anne first came in to see me she had composed herself
remarkably well, but in the next few days I could see that she
was tense. She looked anxious, she spoke in a strained way
and her visits were not restful. She was obviously carrying an
enormous strain, although several close friends gave us
wonderful support and Anne's mother came the next day to
look after everything at home.

We felt that we had to be very careful about communicat-
ing this unexpected news of the spread of cancer into my
liver. It was important for the Christian public to be alerted,
because so many people were praying for me, but at the same
time I was concerned about how my children and my elderly
mother would take it.

We found it more helpful to discuss practical matters
about newsletters and press reports than attempting in any

way to think through the personal and family implications of dying. We were much too vulnerable for that.

Added to that, the busy hospital routine together with the extraordinary cheerfulness of both nurses and patients gave little time for fears and introspection. I felt too weak to read my Bible, apart from a few verses every now and then, and during the three or four days after my operation when I was in the main ward there was constant activity all around me. In the middle of one night, the patient opposite me seemed to lose all control, shouting loudly and demanding to be sent home by taxi immediately. It took the skill and strength of several hospital staff to control him, and I don't think that any of us got much sleep that night.

The worst times for me were at two or three o'clock in the morning. I had preached the gospel all over the world with ringing conviction. I had told countless thousands of people that I was not afraid of death since through Christ I had already received God's gift of eternal life. For years I had not doubted these truths at all. But now the most fundamental questions were nagging away insistently, especially in those long hours of the night. If I was soon on my way to heaven, how real was heaven? Was it anything more than a beautiful idea? What honestly would happen when I died? Did God himself really exist after all? How could I be sure? Indeed, how could I be certain of anything apart from cancer and death? I literally sweated over those questions, and on many occasions woke up with my pyjamas bathed in cold sweat! Never before had my faith been so ferociously attacked.

I remembered those words of Dostoevsky: 'It is not as a child that I believe and confess Jesus Christ. My "hosanna" is born of a furnace of doubt.'

At this point most hospitals have little or nothing to offer apart from drugs. I once asked a leading physician in this country, 'What hope can you offer a man who is dying?' He replied, 'None whatsoever!' During my short stay in Guy's Hospital I chatted several times to doctors and nurses on this theme of death. Here were men and women facing the hard fact of it every day, yet thoroughly confused by it.

In spite of all the marvellous work that continuously takes place in hospitals, those working there are conscious of 'failures'. Some patients are visibly dying. Others, like me, have a 'death sentence' given to them, however kindly. Increasingly doctors are aware of this, and I was undoubtedly impressed with the sensitivity I was shown in Guy's. I felt throughout that they were treating me as a whole person, not only dealing with the disease, and they obviously cared. I could not imagine being better looked after anywhere, and I was full of praise for the combination of their cheerfulness, compassion and efficiency.

My own doubts and questionings did not last for very long, although in the middle of the night I was not always sufficiently awake to counter the sense of fear and foreboding that at times overcame me. Those were times of seeming abandonment – 'My God, my God, why have you forsaken me?' Yet when Christ uttered those terrible words of dereliction on the cross, he was taking upon himself the sin and guilt of the whole world, so that we might be forgiven. We cannot begin to imagine the horror of Christ's spiritual torment, quite apart from the physical and mental agony of crucifixion. But because of his death, I *knew*, in my heart of hearts, that I belonged to God for ever. Nothing could ever separate me from him.

I also knew that, when it comes to facing death, everyone has 'faith'. As I lay there in the early hours of the morning, I knew that I had to trust someone about the future; and there is no one in the history of the world that I would rather trust than Jesus Christ. But there were questions I had to ask myself.

Did Christ really exist? Yes, I had no doubts about that at all. Even Marghanita Laski, a literary critic and a self-confessed atheist, told me when I debated with her on Radio 4 a few years ago, 'I find the Gospels totally convincing as historical documents.' I knew my Christianity was not built on a dream, a religious idea or a fictional character. It was solidly based on a historical person.

Was Christ really the Son of God? Can he be trusted? He certainly made monstrous and outrageous claims for himself if they were not true. Yet everything about his life, ministry and teaching supported his claims. Here surely was the One Person with the right to speak about all the greatest issues of life and death that puzzle us all. He is the Great Consultant. There is every reason why we should trust him. If, on the other hand, we ignore or reject his words, we put ourselves in a far more daring and dangerous position of faith, especially when facing death. Yes, I told myself, I was absolutely sure I could trust Christ for my future.

Did Christ really rise from the dead? Once again, I had for many years sifted through the evidence for this until I was sure beyond any reasonable doubt. The resurrection of Christ was a plain, historical fact – sometimes described as 'the best attested fact in history'.[1] My confidence about the future was not just a psychological prop because I was frightened of death, nor was it clutching at some slender religious straw. Intellectually, I was as convinced as I possibly could be that Christ had risen from the dead, and this was the solid ground for my own future hopes. Death is not the end. There is life after death. Death is only putting out the lamp at the rise of a new dawn.

I am not saying that I never had any problems after that. It would not be true. But in the middle of those nightmare storms, with waves of doubt and fear lashing all around me, I found that my faith was secure on that immovable rock of Christ.

---

[1] I have examined some of the evidence for the resurrection of Christ in *Is Anyone There?*, Hodder and Stoughton, 1979. See also *Man Alive!* by Michael Green, IVP, 1967, or *The Evidence for the Resurrection* by Prof J. N. D. Anderson, IVP, 1950.

7

Encouraging Faith

In no way am I, as a Christian, sheltered from the pains and tears of this world. Sometimes I am crushed and brokenhearted.

My God is Real[1] is a title of a book I wrote some years ago as I tried to express my basic beliefs in God. Intellectually I have been persuaded for years about the reasonableness of the Christian faith, and I was thankful that this faith stood firm when facing the ultimate crisis of a terminal illness and death. God proved himself to be real in the darkness as well as in the light, and I knew that my knowledge of him was growing through this experience.

At the same time I longed for God to speak to me. Although my mind was now clear, my heart needed to be warmed. On this more devotional level I turned to a constant source of inspiration for my faith: the Psalms. In the 150 psalms recorded in the Bible we find almost every human mood and emotion honestly expressed, with a strong confidence in a reigning, living and loving God piercing through the gloom of sickness, suffering, loneliness, depression, fear and death. So many psalms spoke to me personally and became vehicles of communication with God that it is impossible to give more than a few examples. Psalm 30 pinpointed my feelings perfectly, now that I had come through the operation:

[1]Kingsway Publications Ltd, 1970.

> I cried to you for help, O Lord my God,
>> and you healed me;
>> you kept me from the grave.
> I was on my way to the depths below,
>> but you restored my life . . .
> Tears may flow in the night,
>> but joy comes in the morning . . .

Fears often loom large at night-time, when every negative thought can grow hideously out of proportion; but the daylight casts away the shadows and restores a right perspective.

Psalm 91 was one which I had often preached on, but now I found the familiar words personally reassuring:

> Whoever goes to the Lord for safety,
>> whoever remains under the
>> protection of the Almighty,
> can say to him,
>> 'You are my defender and protector.
>> You are my God; in you I trust.'
> He will keep you safe from all hidden dangers
>> and from all deadly diseases.
> He will cover you with his wings;
>> you will be safe in his care;
>> his faithfulness will protect you and
>> defend you.
> You need not fear any dangers at night
>> or sudden attacks during the day
>> or the plagues that strike in the dark
>> or the evils that kill in daylight . . .
> God says, 'I will save those who love
>> me
>> and will protect those who know me
>> as Lord . . .'

I found God's word to be a wonderful protection from all dreadful imaginings. Even on a human level the existence of anxieties and fears can accelerate the disease and hinder the healing process. A number of years ago my local doctor was an agnostic, yet he used to send some of his patients to our church because, he explained to me, he saw that the people who came to him from our church had a quality of peace about them that was a positive influence in healing.

As I read or prayed through those psalms, I was conscious of my tensions unwinding, my fears disappearing, and once again I was aware of the Lord's love surrounding me. I could literally rest in him. In the words of Psalm 139, which is particularly graphic in the *Living Bible*, although not printed as verse, I found an echo for my thoughts:

> You chart the path ahead of me, and tell me where to stop and rest. Every moment you know where I am . . . You both precede and follow me, and place your hand of blessing on my head. This is too glorious, too wonderful to believe! I can *never* be lost to your Spirit! I can *never* get away from my God! If I go up to heaven, you are there; if I go down to the place of the dead, you are there. If I ride the morning winds to the farthest oceans, even there your hand will guide me, your strength will support me. If I try to hide in the darkness, the night becomes light around me. For even darkness cannot hide from God; to you the night shines as bright as day. Darkness and light are both alike to you . . .

Christian evangelists (I am one of them) sometimes speak of the marvellous things that Christ can do for every person. Christ can bring forgiveness, peace, love, freedom, joy, hope, purpose, fulfilment, and so forth. All that is true, as countless people have experienced. But it is not the whole story, as the psalmist discovered, for example in Psalm 73. As I look around it is often the *un*believer who seems to be free and purposeful, confident and assured. In contrast, I often seem to be anxious, unsure, confused, in pain, and sometimes sunk in that dark pit of depression. Although I proclaim that God is real and answers prayer, to be honest he sometimes seems a million miles away and strangely silent to my frightened cries. But I have discovered over the years that although God never promises to save us from suffering, he does promise to be with us in the midst of it and is himself afflicted by it.

The mystics down the centuries have often referred to the 'dark night of the soul'. This describes those periods when God seems strangely silent and absent in spite of personal need. We wonder what he is doing, why he is withholding his presence from us. We pray to him, but the heavens seem as brass and we feel trapped by the prison of our own dark moods. 'The greatest test of a Christian's life is to live with the silence of God,' wrote Bishop Mervyn Stockwood in a letter to me recently. How far can we go on trusting God when we have no experience of his love? Is it enough to take him purely at his word when we feel no reality behind those familiar phrases? It is comforting to see that the psalmist often battled like this:

> How long, O Lord? Wilt thou forget me for ever?
>   How long wilt thou hide thy face from me?
> How long must I bear pain in my soul,
>   and have sorrow in my heart all the day?
> How long shall my enemy be exalted over me?
>
> Psalm 13

Eventually the psalmist knows too much about God and his faithfulness to be crushed for ever:

> But I have trusted in thy steadfast love;
>   my heart shall rejoice in thy salvation.
>
> (verse 5)

Even when all is dark and silent, possibly for months if not years, we can still know that the Lord is there. His word is never broken. His steadfast love never fails.

8

Prayer for Healing

'They are flying over to pray with you and will be here on Wednesday!'

I could hardly believe the news when Anne brought it to me two days after the operation. She was referring to three pastors from California.

Each January, when I am in California as a visiting lecturer at Fuller Theological Seminary, I go whenever possible to a remarkable church called The Vineyard at Yorba Linda, where John Wimber is the main pastor. This church has grown from nothing to 4,000 in four years, and most of those 4,000 have had no links with any church at all before coming to this one. At the time of writing they have no church building of their own.[1] They meet each Sunday in a school gymnasium which looks as unattractively functional as any other big gymnasium. Each Sunday morning a team of men arrive early to roll out some carpets, put up a large number of chairs, erect a small stage and fix some good PA equipment. About half the congregation sit on terraced benches called 'bleachers' (when someone there asked me how I liked the 'bleachers', I thought this must be the name of their music group so I said that they were really great!). Then at the end of each Sunday, everything is put away, ready for school on Monday morning.

What attracts so many to this church? They come in their

[1] They have since moved to a location in Anaheim, California, near Disneyland.

jeans and T-shirts, and superficially nothing could look less like a typical church service. John Wimber, a patriarchial figure with a twinkle in his eye, complete with a bushy beard and an open-necked shirt, leads the service sitting behind an electric piano on which he later rests his Bible and sermon notes. The rest of the music group on the small stage usually consists of three guitarists and a drummer. The whole event is wonderfully relaxed and low-key, with nothing of the showbiz performance common in so many of the big American churches. My first impressions there were dominated by the incredible sense of genuine caring love pervading the entire church, together with a gentle spirit of intimate worship. Although all their songs were quite new to me, I found them easy to learn and anyway was soon caught up in the extraordinary atmosphere of heartfelt praise from the 3,000 who were present.

One of the most powerful attractions of the church, however, is to be found in the 'signs and wonders' which happen at every service. After a sustained time of worship, followed by excellent Bible teaching (usually from John Wimber), those who want to find Christ, or who need healing or other help, are invited into a side room. Probably a hundred or more are counselled and prayed for each week. Remarkable healings take place. And it is not just backaches, headaches and toothaches, although those afflictions are no doubt dealt with too. But the blind receive their sight, the deaf hear, the lame walk, those who are crippled with arthritis are straightened up, those who are barren later give birth to babies, those bound by satanic powers through involvement with the occult are set free. It is not true that *all* who are sick are healed, but a good many are, either immediately or over a period of time during which there is persistent prayer and ministry.

I talked with Mike, an architect, who was so diseased by multiple sclerosis that he could no longer hold his pencil. Of course he had lost his job. At a service in that church God began to heal him over a short space of time, so that now he is fully recovered, working as a professional architect once again.

Last time I was there, a man testified to healing from cancer in the mouth. The chemotherapy had not worked and had been stopped about six months previously. Drastic surgery was now necessary when about half his tongue and three-quarters of his jaw would have to be removed. Although he was not a Christian, the man was brought to this church and God immediately began to heal him. After a few weeks he went back to his doctor and all that could be found of the tumour was some scar tissue.

Similar stories are far too numerous to mention, and some are in the process of being carefully documented at the present time. John Wimber also teaches at Fuller Seminary, and his course on 'Signs and Wonders in Church Growth' is the most popular course ever held there. Seminary professors and other Christian leaders have taken part in this course and testify to the quality and credibility of the teaching.

Over the years I have seen a number of faith-healers at work, and most have left me troubled, if not disillusioned. The strong emotionalism of the meeting, the persuasive pleas for money, the unconfirmed claims of healing – all have left me wary and sceptical. Added to that, for one year in York we prayed fervently for four people who had cancer, three of them young parents. All four died. That rocked our faith in God's power to heal for some time, and we thereafter felt able to pray only for peace in the midst of sickness. Over the years I have been confused and cautious about the whole subject. I have not doubted that God *can* heal, and I have sometimes experienced healing myself, but it has very much been the exception rather than the rule.

What first excited me about John Wimber's church, however, was the indisputable evidence of God's power to heal, coupled with a lot of biblical wisdom and human sanity. They do not have all the answers. They do not guarantee healing. Sometimes they are as puzzled and confused as anyone else. They have their 'failures'. In the first year, when they began to believe and teach that God does heal today, they saw no evidence for it. Those they prayed for remained — sick or grew worse, and even those who prayed for them became sick! But they stuck to it, and eventually healings began to flow.

In the Gospels we see John the Baptist in prison having severe doubts about Jesus being the Messiah after all. 'Are you he who is to come, or shall we look for another?' he asked through two messengers. Dr Luke records, 'In that hour he (Jesus) cured many of diseases and plagues and evil spirits, and on many that were blind he bestowed sight. And he answered them, "Go and tell John what you have *seen and heard* . . ." ' (Luke 7:21f). Here were the signs of the kingdom, the proof of his Messiahship. In the early Church it was the bold preaching of the Gospel together with the demonstration of the power of God, seen visually in the healings that took place, that helped people to believe in Jesus. For example, in Acts 8 we read that Philip went to Samaria to preach Christ. 'And the multitudes with one accord gave heed to what was said by Philip, when they heard him and *saw the signs which he did*. For unclean spirits came out of many who were possessed, crying with a loud voice; and many who were paralysed or lame were healed. So there was much joy in that city.' People need not only to hear about Christ, but to see some evidence of the truth of the Gospel by a demonstration of the Spirit's power.

For a long time I had theoretically believed in the truth of all this, and I had seen *some* healings – together with the striking effect of them – in my own ministry. But never before had I found such a wholesome and powerful healing ministry as at Yorba Linda. Therefore when I was told that John Wimber and two others were flying out to pray with me, I could hardly believe it. Anne and my children, who had seen God's power at work through John and his team in York, were of course thrilled with the news that they were coming. Anne was positively glowing when she told me. Her bright eyes sparkled, and it was the best news she could have brought me.

'John Wimber, Blaine Cook and John McClure are arriving here on Wednesday.'

'That's fantastic!' I replied, hardly able to believe it. The two Johns were both pastors of remarkable churches, and Blaine had a clear, God-given healing ministry. I knew that they were praying for me. But for all three of them to fly over from California seemed incredible. I knew the enormous demands on their time and energy. 'Why bother with me?' I asked myself. 'Why me?' My eyes became moist.

'What did they say?'

'Simply that they loved you and were coming straight over! And they will be here for three days!'

'Well, we must pay for their tickets of course,' I said. 'If we got all our savings together I think we can manage it. Where are they staying?'

'They're booking rooms in a hotel because they don't want to be a burden on anyone!'

I was astonished by such an expression of love. Although their wide experience with healing obviously gave me fresh encouragement and hope, I think it was this tangible expression of caring love which did more for me than anything else. How often had I been too busy to see a sick person when it meant only a couple of hours out of my day! Here were three extremely busy men flying across the Atlantic and spending almost a week of their time – to visit me!

When Anne left, I was filled with praise that God loved me so much – a love wonderfully expressed through his worldwide family. I opened my Bible and read several psalms of thanksgiving and praise. However long or short my life might be, nothing was more profound or important than knowing that God loved me. I was almost ready to die immediately that I might know the fulfilment of God's love in heaven. But I did not think that these friends were flying over just for my funeral!

On the Tuesday after my operation, the various tubes were

removed out of my body, which I found slightly unpleasant but I was thankful to be less tied down.

'Sister,' I asked, 'is there any chance of my going back into the side room, since the three pastors are arriving tomorrow and want to spend time praying with me?' I had already talked to the Sister and nurses about my friends and their remarkable healing ministry. I knew the ward staff were at least intrigued, and all had been sad about the discovery of cancer in my liver.

'Yes, that should be possible,' she replied.

I hoped there would be no relapse. That evening, when the house doctor was in the ward, I had a persistent attack of hiccups which simply would not go away.

'Put a tube down his throat,' said the doctor. The shock treatment of this had the desired result: my hiccups vanished instantly.

The next day I was wheeled into the side room and tidied up for the normal doctor's round. They had only just left the room when I heard a familiar and welcome voice.

'Hi there, David. How yer doin'?'

'John!' I said, almost jumping out of my bed. 'How wonderful to see you. And Blaine! And John! I can hardly believe it!'

'Well, you don't look as if you're exactly dying!' said John with a twinkle. 'You look great!'

'You sure do,' said Blaine and John McClure.

I thought it was a bit of flattery, since I had lost a lot of weight and was not exactly the picture of health. But my eyes sparkled with joy at their presence. I have seldom met with such genuinely loving and caring people as those three. They had just flown into Heathrow after a sleepless night, and had come straight from the airport to the hospital. I knew that they loved me and that they had flown over because they believed that God wanted to heal me.

We chatted about the events of the last two weeks, and they explained that this was only a preliminary visit. After a good night's sleep they would return tomorrow to pray for me. But as we talked, they sensed the power of God coming upon them, so they began to pray. They praised God for his presence with us, for his authority over life and death, and they prayed against the spirit of unbelief, fear and death that was pervading the room.

After some time of praise and worship, Blaine became aware of the activity of the Holy Spirit, and laid hands on my abdomen. The three of them went on praying, cursing the cancer in the name of Christ, commanding it to wither, and then they claimed God's healing in my body. If this seems a little strange, it is no more so than the incidents in the Gospels where Jesus rebuked a fever (Luke 4:38f) or cursed a fig-tree (Mark 11:12–25). The power of God was certainly with him.

I felt a tremendous surge of heat as well as vibrations in my body, and I knew that God was at work. This went on for half an hour or more, and we all had no doubt that God was with us.

'That was quite a time!' said John Wimber (as indeed it was). 'We had no intention of praying for you until tomorrow, but it seemed that God just stepped in! In fact I sense that the work we came over to do has now been done. Anyway, we'll come again tomorrow to see how you are doing.'

As they left, I was undoubtedly 'doing' very well. I was bursting with praise. It was as though I had been lifted up into the presence of God, bathed in his glory and enveloped in his love. The light of Christ banished any remaining areas of doubt and fear, and I knew that, whatever the future might hold, I was safe in his hands. When a friend came to visit me later that day I said 'I feel five hundred times better.' I gather that even my appearance had changed quite dramatically.

When Anne arrived we were obviously both overjoyed.

'Have you found out how much their tickets cost?' I asked.

'They won't take a penny from us,' she replied. 'In fact they've brought us a generous gift for your recuperation.'

It was hard to take it in, but thankfully we accepted this sign of their love.

The two Johns and Blaine came back on the Thursday and Friday. Mostly we talked and laughed. They were convinced that the main work was now done, and there was no need for further lengthy sessions of prayer. Certainly they did pray again, with great authority in the name of Christ – so loudly at times that I thought that everyone in the ward knew exactly what was being said – and again they laid their hands on me to encourage my faith. None of this had the same unexpected touch of power as on the first occasion, but I was sure that God was, through them, continuing the work that he had begun.

John Wimber warned me that sometimes, in his experience, a tumour will grow after a time of prayer, until it begins to wither and die.

'It might well be that the next scan or two will reveal cancer in your liver, a cancer that is growing. But I believe that the root of it has now been cut. And soon it will begin to die.'

When they eventually departed to fly back to Los Angeles, I was left with an overwhelming sense of God, and my whole being wanted to worship him. So I relaxed on my bed and did just that.

9

Enjoying God

Two friends of mine had lent me their stereo tape-recorder together with headphones, and I found that my faith in God's love and power to heal was stirred not only by the psalms and other Bible passages I was reading but by the songs of praise I was listening to. John Wimber had brought me a cassette of one of their evening services, and its spirit of worship gloriously refreshed me. It was like having a relaxing bath or shower! Anne brought me several other cassettes, and I was also sent the latest one from St Michael-le-Belfrey in York called *Come and Worship*. That opened with my favourite song from Psalm 16 'For You Are My God', and I found that the whole cassette seemed to fill my being with praise.

With headphones over my ears, my eyes closed, a beatific smile on my face, and my hands sometimes raised in worship, I must have looked a strange sight! So it was not surprising when the nurse on night-duty looked through the small glass window into my room, saw this apparition and then rushed in to take my temperature and pulse! All was well. In spite of my recent operation and a bleak prognosis, I was transported with joy. The love of God seemed to fill the whole room and I was profoundly aware of his presence. I knew deep within my spirit that nothing could be more wonderful than being perfectly with him in heaven and seeing him face to face, although we had just prayed for healing in order to be on earth for a little bit longer!

At that moment, however, it was not the length of life that was important but its quality; and in the Bible *eternal life* refers to the quality of life, not simply duration. I am not sure that words like *duration* mean very much in the next world anyway since time is a human limitation. God is outside time; and *eternal life* means life with God and with his Son Jesus Christ. This begins on this earth when we commit our lives to Christ, but comes to completion after death. Often I have experienced a foretaste of heaven during times of worship when, in company with God's people, we have been 'lost in wonder, love and praise'. All worries and fears have paled into insignificance. The consuming impression is that God is in our midst, 'inhabiting the praises of his people'.

Churches throughout the world that have seen God at work in unusual power, often in the area of healing, all stress the absolute importance of worship. All too often our faith is earth-bound and we find it hard to believe that God can do anything that our minds cannot explain. It is only as we spend time worshipping God, concentrating on the nature of his Person, especially his greatness and love, that our faith begins to rise. Like a plane soaring through the dark rain-clouds into the fresh beauty of the sunshine, so our faith rises, stimulated by worship and by the new vision of God that worship brings, until we begin to believe that God can work in ways that may be beyond our present understanding.

It is significant that the Church was born in praise. When the Holy Spirit fell on the disciples on the Day of Pentecost, their immediate response was to worship God for all his wonderful works – and they did this in languages given to them by the Spirit. It is not surprising, therefore, that in the same chapter we read that 'many wonders and signs were done through the apostles', and in the next chapter a well-known cripple is healed through Peter and John. Indeed throughout those early chapters of Acts we find this constant blend of worship and wonders, praise and power. An interesting paraphrase by Strong of Psalm 50:23 reads: 'To him that uses praise over and over again, enough to make a trodden path, will I show the deliverance of God.' There are countless examples in the Bible and in Christian biography where a sustained time of praise prepares the way for the Lord to demonstrate his power.

It is a sad commentary on the life of the Church in this country today that worship is often sterile and dull, and at the same time the level of faith to be found in many congregations is dismally low. The two factors almost inevitably go together. And if in God's goodness there is a resurgence of a vital faith, almost certainly it will be accompanied by – or more likely preceded by – a fresh spirit of praise. John Wesley used to tell his disciples to preach faith until they got it. By this he meant that as we proclaim God's word, so our faith in God will grow. The same is true when we worship God.

For many years I had both known and taught the power of praise. During my seventeen years in York I had sought to develop various expressions of worship in our church, and have always tried to stress the vital relevance of this in Festivals of Praise we have led in many different parts of the world. All too often I have attended dreary services when I have come away spiritually more dead than alive. Any thinking person, searching for a personal faith, might well conclude that surely God was not in that place. This is a travesty of the vibrant worship that should always be there when God's people come together to praise his name. The format or liturgy of the service is not a priority for me (although I happen to like the Anglican services), but I long to be in a place where the worship is *alive*. The Jewish festivals in Old Testament days were full of music, singing and dancing, and we can understand why the psalmist said, 'I was glad when they said to me, "Let us go to the house of the Lord!" ' (Psalm 122:1). Those festivals were such exuberant, colourful and joyful events that the sound of thousands of people praising God could be heard for miles around.

I have been privileged to take part in many hundreds of similar occasions which have been marked, not only by an exultant note of celebration, but by a profound sense of God's presence. On such occasions I have seen agnostics and even atheists becoming aware of God and brought to know him and worship him for themselves – essentially through the praises of his people. Constantly, too, I have seen the faith of true believers rise above their own personal problems in such an atmosphere of praise. I have met many who have been healed of illnesses, even major ones such as multiple sclerosis and cancer, through the power of the Spirit of God released in praise. Lives have been significantly changed, stubborn wills broken, relationships restored, faith and hope renewed – all resulting from joyful and intimate worship.

The most common word for worship in the New Testament comes sixty-six times. It could be translated 'I come towards to kiss'. God is love, and he wants us to respond to him in love. He wants us to enjoy a love-relationship with him, expressed partly through praise. People today need to know that God loves them as individuals, just as they are, with all their faults and failings. Often the common feeling is that God, if he exists at all, is a million miles away, aloof, distant, far removed from our personal needs, seemingly silent to all our cries for help. Those who believe in him are usually afraid of him, unsure of him and only too ready to believe that sickness is some sort of punishment for past sins. Comparatively few know, deep down within their hearts, that God really loves them more than they could ever begin to imagine. However, when we 'come towards to kiss' by opening our hearts to him in worship, we are able to receive his love poured into our hearts by the Holy Spirit (Romans 5:5). Whatever our feelings may be (and feelings are fickle) we become *aware* of God's personal love for us. Interestingly the Christian mystics of the past have often referred to God's Spirit as his kiss, so that being filled with his Spirit is simply allowing ourselves to be kissed by God. Here we have the intimacy of love in our relationship with God that we read about so often in the Bible, notably in the Psalms and in the Song of Solomon.

> O God, thou art my God,
>   I seek thee,
>   my soul thirsts for thee;
> my flesh faints for thee,
>   . . .
>
> Because thy steadfast love is
>   better than life,
>   my lips will praise thee . . .
>
> (Psalm 63:1, 3)

As we 'come towards to kiss' in worship, so God comes afresh to us with the kiss of his Spirit.

It is one thing mentally to believe the statement 'God loves you'; it is quite another to have a deep certainty of that within my heart and spirit. Yet that certainty is so crucial in times of crisis: a quiet, settled conviction and faith. I have found that such faith is encouraged (and it needs daily encouragement) partly by meditating on God's word of love in the scriptures, partly by the expression of God's love through caring Christian friends, but perhaps mostly by the inward experiencing of God's love through sensitive and joyful worship.

Never has the reality of such worship meant so much to me as during this time when I have had to realise the basic truth that my life is literally in God's hands. The apostle John once wrote that 'there is no fear in love, but perfect love casts out fear' (1 John 4:18). When we are quite sure that God loves us and have his perfect love within our hearts, all fears about pain, sickness and death must vanish. There is no room for them. As soon as we lose that conscious awareness of his love, even when in our minds we may still know it to be true, those fears may return to haunt and disturb.

Faith is a living thing. It is like a plant that needs constant feeding. If we take daily and active steps to nourish our faith we shall find ourselves kept in God's peace and love, whatever storms may be raging around us. When we are feeling ill, it is often the task of others to pray for us and to bring God's love to us. It is their faith that counts, not ours. But one way or another, we need to find God's love and stay resting in it. Nothing is more important than that.

10

Letters Galore!

'We love you very much and know the tender arms of Jesus will enfold you at all times. Constantly praying and praising God for you both.'

That telegram from Edmonton in Canada, arriving just before my operation, was typical of the deluge of cables, letters, cards and messages that flooded in during the following weeks. Over a thousand arrived in the first month, and another thousand or so after that. They came from people of all walks of life and from all over the world. I literally wept when reading the expressions of love and deep tender concern from such a multitude of people, many of whom I never knew personally.

I was profoundly moved when I heard that thousands of Christians in Zimbabwe were praying for me – and I have never been to Zimbabwe! I was astonished to discover that Catholic and Protestant terrorists who had come to Christ were joining together to pray for me in a prison in Northern Ireland: I had several marvellous letters from a former IRA and INLA leader who was on hunger strike in the Maze Prison for fifty-five days and who, having come to the very threshold of death, had turned to Christ and is now serving the Lord 'with a glowing witness', as a mutual friend describes it. This ex-terrorist wrote long letters to encourage my faith and went on to say, 'It is my hope that we who have been through violent organisations can come together in Jesus to spread the message of love and reconciliation in a hate-filled society.' He spoke of over eighty prisoners who had found Jesus, and ended with these words: 'David, my brother in Jesus . . . May God's love and peace which passes all understanding be with you and all your loved ones. Your brother and friend in Jesus . . .'

I was humbled to receive numerous letters from church leaders from almost all denominations throughout the world, including the Archbishops of Canterbury and York and many other bishops from all over the Anglican Communion. Messages of love, concern and the promise of prayer came from almost everywhere: from Singapore to South Africa, from Israel to Argentina, from the United States to Yugoslavia, from New Zealand to Switzerland, from Sweden to South India, from Australia to Canada, and of course from all over Great Britain. Never before have I felt so much a part of the world-wide Body of Christ. The reality of being 'all one in Christ' came home to me with astonishing force. For years I had declared in the words of the Apostles' Creed, 'I believe in the Holy Spirit, the holy catholic Church, the communion of saints . . .' The deep sense of belonging not only to God but also to his family all over the world and throughout all ages brought to me an incredible sense of security and peace.

I had always heard that Christians in communist prisons, or suffering elsewhere for their faith, had thought much about their solidarity with all those in Christ, regardless of denomination, race or colour. Some of my greatest support and most sensitive expressions of love came from Roman Catholic friends, who probably stirred up my faith in the love of Christ more than anyone. I was also particularly touched by the warmth of God's love expressed by Christians of all races in South Africa. Many letters began in the same way, 'Dear David, you won't know me but . . .' Then would follow a moving account of how that person had found Christ through my preaching or writing, or else had been specifically helped by me although I had never known it until my illness.

I remember once being challenged by the question, 'Have you ever thanked those who have been an encouragement to you in the past? Have you ever written to your teacher, doctor, nurse, social worker, employer, vicar, or whoever, and told them how they had helped you at some important moment in your life?' Often I can be critical. I complain readily enough, and do not easily forget those times when I have been hurt or let down. However I realise that I can encourage people when I take the trouble to thank those who have done something positive for me. Prompted by my illness, and perhaps with the thought that I might not be on this earth for much longer, I wrote several letters to this effect and received many more. I was able to praise God that he had been able to use my feeble and faltering efforts to touch other people's lives.

What I found particularly valuable were fairly brief re-assurances of love and prayer. I could not cope with lengthy letters, with a few special exceptions from those I knew very well; but I found great comfort in short affirmative comments such as this one from a wonderful Christian leader and a close personal friend: 'David, my brother, you are loved, appreciated, much prayed for, greatly needed, and we do not "accept" your illness. "God is greater." ' Such letters take only a minute or two to write and bring inspiration out of all proportion to their length.

An ex-heroin addict promised, 'You can be assured of my constant prayers and of my love for you as a sister in Christ,' and she enclosed a moving poem she had written about the time when Jesus had found her in the midst of her addiction:

> When I gave up and prayed to die,
>   you breathed in me your life;
> When I screamed in the darkness,
>   your light shone down on my heart . . .

A retired university professor wrote about the grief he experi-enced with the news of my illness: '(It) has hurt and distres-sed me . . . The stark reality of it wounds me . . . Dear David, I know God has been with you all your life, and he will sustain you now to strengthen and restore you, whom he loves so dearly . . .'

David Pawson, the well-known preacher and a personal friend wrote about the time when his wife was diagnosed as having cancer:

> It was then that we discovered the difference between being *willing* to go to heaven while *wanting* to stay on earth (for the sake of family, friends, etc) – and *wanting* to go to heaven while being *willing* to stay on earth for others' sake (which was Paul's position in Philippians 1). We found there was great release in getting through to Paul's position – and that only then could we approach the question of healing in an objective way. We simply told the Lord that *if* he had more work on earth for my wife to do then he knew what he had to do about it. He had and he did, bless him!

I found that especially helpful. I was certainly willing to go to heaven, but I very much wanted to be around for a little longer, at least until my children were grown-up and able to look after themselves and Anne. Knowing how much I missed my own father when he died (I was ten), I did not want them to go through the same difficulties. However, as I continued to abandon everything, including my family, to the Lord, and as I continued to worship him and reflect on his word in the Bible, so I found myself (at least sometimes, to be honest) genuinely *wanting* to be with him in heaven, but willing to stay on earth in order to serve him and others here. It was an attitude of great security, although I realised it should be the constant position of every Christian. In theory it had been mine and I had always looked forward to heaven. But when the crunch came, I was not too sure!

Some letters, inevitably, were less helpful, most of them coming from complete strangers. It is amazing how many I received which went something like this: 'Dear David (or Canon Watson, or Rev, or Sir), You won't know me. I'm

sorry to hear you have cancer. My husband got cancer last
year and he died last month . . .' Then followed page after
page of almost illegible writing giving details of all the painful
therapy the husband had to go through, all the traumas
surrounding death and all the problems the family had to
suffer.

However, these were vastly more helpful than some letters
I received. One person wrote with conviction about the after
life urging me to 'find a reliable clairaudient medium,
through whom you could converse sometimes with your dear
wife'!

I could not but smile at the thought that some well-
meaning writers had me effectively dead and buried a little
before my time! A few letters read like obituaries, and I
remembered Mark Twain's comment when he saw, to his
surprise, his own obituary in the national papers: 'The report
of my death was an exaggeration.' Shortly after I had left
hospital someone rang up a Bible College in this country to
ask about my progress. When told I had 'gone home', the
rumour of my supposed death caused no little stir in some
parts of the country.

A number of letters never reached me at all. My wife and
secretary carefully screened all the correspondence before
letting me see it, and wisely destroyed all the really unhelpful
stuff, however good the intentions were on the part of the
senders. One man wrote to Anne saying that his own wife
had died, even though she believed to the end that God
would heal her. However, he went on happily to say, he had
now married again and his second marriage was unbeliev-
ably wonderful. They were blissfully happy! The next day
poor Anne got another letter from this man's second wife to
confirm how glorious it now was. So Anne must not be
discouraged. She could look forward to good, if not much
better, things to come! (I cannot record the words accurately
since both letters were promptly destroyed. No doubt encouragement was intended, but neither letter was the height
of sensitivity when I was fighting for my life!) Both Anne and

I were beginning to learn that, at all stages of recovery, and especially just after an operation, the emotions are vulnerable. Negative emotions can hinder the healing process and even encourage disease, so should be avoided as far as possible.

Fears and doubts continued to afflict me from time to time, partly because of the confusion we were in, intensified by the thousands of letters that arrived. I sensed that a friend of mine hit the nail on the head when he wrote that 'the thing that is holding back complete healing is a combination of fears and doubts within David . . . Stop asking for complete healing and ask for complete trust.' I observed for a time that when I talked about certain aspects of my illness or expectation of healing, some nervous symptoms were apparent: I became breathless or went often to the loo. Although outwardly I seemed fairly peaceful about the present and future, there was still a battle between faith and fear raging within. I noted with care, therefore, the advice of a Christian doctor who wrote:

It is easier to prepare for healing than for parting. But to fail to prepare for parting is to leave a bitter legacy for those we love. David, if it should be that your disease progresses, make time for Anne, Fiona and Guy, to say thank you and to ask forgiveness and to say goodbye.

It was not what I wanted to read, but it was realistic. After all, the time comes for each one of us to die. It is our only future certainty. I did not think that God's time had yet come -- but one day it will. Nothing is more important than our relationships as that day approaches: first and foremost our relationship with God, but also our relationships with others, especially our family. In our busy western society, we put too much emphasis on work, achievements, money and success, invariably at the expense of relationships. Above all, if God allowed me a peaceful rather than a violent death, I wanted time to say goodbye to my family. For those in Christ it is only *au revoir*. We shall meet each other again.

Visitors also were screened so that only a strictly limited number of helpful people were allowed to come. I heard of someone who was hospitalised after a severe road accident, and who subsequently had such a stream of well-meaning visitors that in the first month he had only half an hour alone with his wife. Michael Griffiths, the wise Christian leader who told me this story, urged me 'to guard your privacy and time with your family'. For a good many weeks after the operation I was physically weak and grew tired very easily, so that a careful rationing of callers was important.

Some people found it hard to accept that I did not want to see them at that time. Hilary had to be extremely firm and yet tactful on the telephone on many occasions. I do not doubt that the individuals concerned desired only to cheer me up and to pray with me, but they seemed unable to understand that I was exhausted and that Anne was under considerable strain. The last thing we wanted was to see one person after another, answering the same questions, talking over the same issues, and listening to much conflicting advice. We had to be ruthless about this for a good many weeks. Obviously in hospital I loved seeing Anne and Fiona (Guy being away at school), and I was greatly helped by *brief* visits from close friends who chatted for a short time, read a verse or two from the Bible and then prayed for me. It is what I had done for hundreds of people in the past, but it was good to be on the receiving end for a change. I found two or three visits from John and Diana Collins especially helpful. They sometimes came on Sunday evenings after their services at Holy Trinity Brompton were over. John read to me a promise from the Bible and both prayed. In one sense it was all very simple, but I was aware of their concern and love, and my faith was always encouraged as a result.

There were also a few surprises. I was quietly dozing on my bed one afternoon when the Sister of the ward came in with a young woman in her early twenties. In my sleepy state

I thought she was an actress who used to be a member of my team, so I said 'How lovely to see you!' and gave her a loving kiss on the cheek. When she sat down on my bed, however, I suddenly realised my mistake. As far as I knew I had never seen this girl before in my life! I was too confused to admit my error, and she looked a little surprised as well. Later I discovered that she was the nurse who had taken me to the theatre for the operation, and she had simply come back to find out how I was getting on.

'Lord Ingleby has just rung up,' said the Sister one day. 'He and Lady Masham are coming to see you tomorrow afternoon.'

I was astonished. It was not so much the privilege of being visited by two members of the House of Lords that amazed me; it was the fact that both Lord Ingleby and Lady Masham were confined to wheel chairs (one through illness, the other through an accident), and it seemed incredible that both should take the considerable trouble of coming to my room in Guy's Hospital. But they made it! They bundled themselves into a taxi outside the House of Lords, struggled out again at the hospital, and then wheeled themselves through seemingly miles of corridors until they sailed into my ward.

'How wonderful of you both to come,' I said. And I was so pleased to see them.

'You fight it! You fight it!' said Sue Masham.

'I have every intention of doing so,' I replied, and went on to describe what had happened so far. I knew that both Martin Ingleby and Sue Masham had been great fighters themselves with indomitable courage, not only as far as their own disabilities were concerned, but in their many battles on behalf of the sick and disabled.

Martin was particularly intrigued by the visit of the American pastors, and I told them all about it.

Eventually they left for their separate engagements that evening. As they propelled themselves down the corridor I felt immensely happy. Here were two lovely people who knew all about suffering and facing uncertain futures, but who were undoubtedly winning the daily battle, and with enormous cheerfulness.

On another day I was both amazed and humbled to learn that, together with numerous gatherings for prayer concerning my healing, a special 'healing eucharist' was being held for me in our old church in York, with Bishop Morris Maddocks taking part. Not only that, but on the same evening thirteen other healing eucharists were being held for the same purpose in different centres throughout the country, and I was overjoyed to hear later on how special the services had been for a great many people. Quite apart from the benefit that I was receiving from all this, I learnt of others being healed, broken relationships being restored, and fresh commitments being made to Christ. If nothing else happened, it seemed that my illness had helped all sorts of people to examine carefully their relationship with God and the priorities in their lives. Almost every day brought unusual and encouraging news like this, and I was astonished by the love and concern of so many people, many of whom were strangers to me yet belonging to God's great family of Christians of all traditions.

I was fortunate to be in an excellent ward, which was run by an attractive, gracious, hard-working and extremely efficient Sister, Jill Purkiss, who won the respect of all the nurses and patients alike. Although I have never enjoyed hospitals, I respect the enormous amount of good work that goes on in them, and I could not imagine being in a better ward anywhere. I was able to relax with confidence, and could accept very gratefully the constant care and attention that they gave me. I am sure that this, together with the huge volume of prayer and love, helped to get me on my feet surprisingly quickly.

To begin with, it was rather a struggle. I had been watching fellow-patients staggering slowly down the corridor and returning a few moments later as though they had just finished the marathon. But with my incision from my navel downwards, I was bent double, and on my first excursion one circuit round my bed was all that I could manage! Steadily this lengthened through the gentle and encouraging persuasion of the physiotherapist, and within a few days I was walking briskly – or rather shuffling determinedly – as often as I could in order to rebuild my strength.

The great day came when the stitches were removed, and I knew that good progress was being made. The only minor setback was when I was given an aperient. It had a devastating effect on me. As soon as I left the loo, I had to rush back as fast as my feeble legs could carry me, desperately hoping that another patient hadn't got there first!

'I simply will *not* take any more of that "crippling gravel" you are giving me,' I said defiantly. The 'gravel' was a form of concentrated bran. Quite lethal!

Then the bliss of my first bath! As I lay there, soaking in the water, I felt like a civilised being once again. However short my life would be – I was going to relish all that I found enjoyable, including a bath.

The day came to leave. As I dressed I was conscious of still being extremely weak and a little unsure as to how I – or my family – would cope with my being at home again. But it was certainly good to be going, even though my time in Guy's had been much happier and less painful than I had anticipated, due to the excellent medical care I had received.

Anne came with Teddy Saunders in his car, and they carried the piles of cards and letters that had been flowing in. I felt a little faint and distinctly cold as we wound our way through the busy London streets. The major battle of my operation had now been fought and largely won. The question facing me now was how far I could trust God for the healing of terminal cancer. Various forms of treatment might possibly prolong my life a little – often with considerable reduction of the quality of life. But would I be healed?

11

What is Reality?

With a clear, reasoned and (I thought) strong belief in God, why was my mind finding it hard at times to accept that God was healing my cancer in the liver? I had argued and debated about the reality of God for nearly thirty years, and was intellectually more convinced than ever, as well as seeing him at work in my own life and in the lives of countless others – sometimes in dramatic ways. If God could change the hearts of violent, hate-filled terrorists, re-making them into loving, caring Christians (as I had several times witnessed), the healing of a physical disease should be comparatively simple. Why then did I fluctuate between faith and doubt?

I knew that my problem was primarily cultural. Together with the vast majority of people living in the West, I was bound by the western scientific world-view.

A *world-view* is the way in which we view or consider the world. It is 'a set of presuppositions (or assumptions) which we hold (consciously or unconsciously) about the basic make-up of our world.'[1] For most people the real world is that which we can see, touch, measure or understand. For us, this is not only reality; it is *total* reality. It is what science can explain and what our rational minds can grasp. We are instinctively suspicious of anything beyond this, and tend to dismiss all unexplainable phenomena as misleading or false. On the whole we do not believe in 'ghosties and ghoulies and things that go bump in the night'. In our sophisticated

[1] *The Universe Next Door*, James Sire, American IVP.

twentieth-century society we are instinctively cautious of the mysterious realm of the spirit.

In the eighteenth century, Immanuel Kant maintained that all knowledge was acquired from a combination of what we can reason with our minds and experience with our senses. God, he said, was therefore unknowable. Kant was not the first to say this, but millions of people in the west today hold roughly this position and are agnostic about God's existence and about spiritual realities.

The widespread assumption is that anything that cannot be proved scientifically is either meaningless and not worthy of serious consideration, or at least suspect and well avoided. Statements about God are increasingly dismissed as unfounded superstition, and attempts to heal the sick through faith are opposed (sometimes fiercely) as medically dangerous. We have given the medical profession authority over life and death, and only through the progress of medical science do we hope to find both the cause and cure of disease. Everything outside the strict boundaries of science is viewed as dangerous and false. This is the western scientific worldview.

It is worth stressing at this point that there are defined limits to the scope of science. Science essentially is descriptive in that it describes what can be seen or measured, but it cannot interpret what it sees or measures. For example, science cannot comment on the statement 'Jane was healed through prayer'; it cannot say whether that is true or false. It can only investigate the statement 'Jane was healed'. It is entirely outside the field of science to determine the significance of the words 'through prayer'. The mistake arises if we assume that such words can have no significance at all. In the same way science cannot comment on the beauty of a sunset or on the love between a man and a woman. Such words as 'beauty' and 'love' are outside the language of science, but that in no way diminishes their reality. I heard of an entry in a communist textbook which defined a *kiss* as 'the approach of two pairs of lips with reciprocal transmission of

microbes and carbon dioxide'. Tell that to a couple of lovers!
As valuable as science undoubtedly is, there are vast stretches of reality which lie beyond its borders.

In spite of this rather obvious fact, the scientific world-
view has thoroughly permeated our western society and,
almost inevitably, has influenced much of the Christian
Church. Although orthodox Christians fully accept the healings, miracles and resurrection of Jesus, as recorded in the
Gospels, many have the greatest difficulty in believing that
similar healings can happen today. Some take the position
that such signs and wonders were only for the apostolic
period in order to establish the truth of the Gospel.

Other Christians accept theoretically that God can heal
today, since his essential character never changes, but in
practice they assume that, although certain extraordinary
happenings occurred when Jesus walked this earth, God's
healing ministry has now been transferred to the medical
profession. No doubt much of it has. We thank God for this.
It is therefore the Church's calling, say some, merely to bring
God's comfort and peace to the sick, in order to encourage
the normal healing process, but not to expect anything more
in answer to the prayer of faith.

A few well-known Christians wrote to me offering no hope
of healing in this life, but reassured me that heaven was not
such a bad place for me to look forward to! 'This life isn't all
there is!' said someone. That is wonderfully true. A Christian
can have a gloriously positive hope for the future, come what
may, since heaven will literally be *heaven*. Nothing could be
more perfect than that, and on numerous occasions I have
felt that I can hardly wait to get there! Nevertheless I was not
sure that my time to leave this world had yet come.

Science is undoubtedly a wonderful part of God's creation.
At the same time God is bigger than science, and we should
not reject various aspects of his nature or working that lie
outside our present scientific knowledge. Paul, in Romans 1,
shows the foolishness of those who suppress the truth of God
that can be known and who 'worship and serve what God has

created instead of the Creator himself.' This is exactly what we have done with science. Instead of seeing science as an invaluable servant for the benefit of mankind, we have elevated it into an object for awe and worship. It controls our minds. It limits our faith. It dictates our understanding. It is the master of our lives and we have become its slaves. What science says is true. No other truth is permissible.

The fact remains, however, that our total human understanding is both finite and limited. God, if he exists at all, is an infinite God and infinitely greater than the finite circle of our understanding. We would all be incurably agnostic unless God had broken through that circle in ways that we can understand. It is the Christian conviction that God has done precisely that: through *creation*, which shows us the power of God, through *conscience*, which shows us the goodness of God, through the *scriptures*, which show us the wisdom and justice of God, but supremely through *Jesus of Nazareth*, who was the Son of God and the living revelation of God on earth. Here is something our minds can grasp concerning the truth of God. 'He who has seen me has seen the Father,' said Jesus. If we want to know what God is like, we start with Jesus. Even here we cannot know the total truth of an infinite God, for that would be impossible for our finite mind, but we can know truths that are important. We may not understand how he healed the sick, nor how the disciples went out and did the same. Certainly the disciples did not understand for they were frequently amazed by the power of Christ; but they went on healing as Christ had commissioned them, for many years to come.

After all, can an infinite personal God possibly be limited by the logic of science? Science may well be a description of the usually ordered nature of God's creation, but that in no way precludes the possibility of his working in extraordinary ways. Christians believe that he has certainly done so many times in the history of God's people, especially during the three years' ministry of Jesus. Why can he not do it again? Although it is a Christian belief that every good gift comes

from God and therefore we should thank God for the wonderful discoveries of medical science (I would not be alive
without this), it would be a profound mistake to assume that
God today can do no more than this. Christians believe that
God forgives all our sins, offers us a new life in Christ and
promises us a place in heaven. If such beliefs are true (and I
have good reasons for believing that they are) these are
staggering achievements of God's grace in our sinful world.

Paul once summarised the heart of the matter like this:
'When someone becomes a Christian he becomes a brand
new person inside. He is not the same any more. A new life
has begun!' (2 Corinthians 5:17, *Living Bible*). This miracle of
'new birth' is a fact I have constantly witnessed over the last
thirty years in countless people. Many Christians maintain
that this is the greatest miracle of all, since there is no other
power on earth that can change human nature. I agree with
them. Why then did I find it so difficult to believe in God's
power to heal physically? If I accepted the spiritual and
eternal blessings of the Gospel, why were the physical and
temporal blessings so much harder to believe? What sort of a
God did I really believe in? Is he a God who can work within
us only what *cannot* be seen and proved? If I genuinely believe
that God intervenes in our lives by guiding us, strengthening
us and steadily transforming us, why can he not heal us as
well? I could see that there was an inconsistency here in my
faith – almost an unconscious 'double-think'. The reason
could be only my bondage to the scientific world-view.

Eastern and Third World countries which are not so
bound to this view have no such problems with healings, and
significantly it is in these underprivileged places that we find
signs and wonders occurring today with New Testament
profusion. Most of these countries could benefit considerably
from the achievements of science that we take for granted in
our own culture, but it is an age-old principle that God has
'chosen those who are poor in the world to be rich in faith and
heirs of the kingdom' (James 2:5). They have no difficulty in
believing that God works today as he did through Jesus and

the apostles. Maybe no one has told them anything different. They expect healing to be part of the good news of the Gospel, and so they see God's power at work in ways that would astonish the scepticism of the West. Sometimes their beliefs may be confused with superstition and primitive rites. However, total reality for them includes the activity of both natural and supernatural forces, and with a clear conversion to Christ they expect God to heal the sick in answer to the prayer of faith. Often he does.

In all this, it would be foolish to imagine science as an enemy of faith. The Christian believes that all good things ultimately come from God, and undoubtedly we enjoy a multitude of 'good things' as a result of science, not least medical science. We should thank God for everything which helps to prevent or cure disease.

What is needed is not a rejection of science in favour of faith, but a widening of our world-view. We need an alternative world-view which embraces humbly all that science can offer and yet appreciates that there is more to come. It is like seeing the world with an extra dimension which in no way denies the other dimensions but presents another perspective. This is what Jesus meant by the Kingdom of God.

12

Back at Home

I had been warned that going home after a major operation is not always easy. Outside the routine and facilities of a hospital it takes time to adjust to the more usual environment of home life. But I was not ready for some of the battles we had to face.

I was naturally overjoyed to be home again, but felt extremely cold after the considerable warmth of the hospital. It was January 26th, and doubtless the accumulated shock to my system of the past few weeks also contributed to the feeling of being frozen. I went to a small guest-room at the top of the house since it was nearer to the loo than our own bedroom, and there was also a better chance that Anne would sleep even if my nights were disturbed.

What was particularly frustrating was attempting to get my bowels to function properly again. I had eaten nothing for ten days in hospital, and then only small amounts of food after that. Obviously I had not been to the loo for some time, so I was given some aperient to get me started again. Every aperient had a violent reaction on my insides, and for weeks I would spend roughly two hours a day (or night) in the loo. It was the only unheated room in the house and not exactly the height of comfort, but it was exceedingly necessary! Looking back on it all, I can laugh at the earthy way my whole life seemed to be dominated by my bowels! I felt just like an old car: either *won't go* or *can't stop*. It was hard to think about anything else, and certainly my days and nights focused on my either far-too-successful or totally-unsuccessful trips to the loo.

Eventually I triumphed over the problem. I bought myself a cheap cassette recorder with headphones, and during the day-time I listened to an extremely helpful series of cassettes on healing, given by John Wimber; whilst at night, with concentration at a considerably lower level at two o'clock in the morning, I listened to worship cassettes. In this way, and in this somewhat unusual posture, I listened to more than forty teaching cassettes and numerous hours of praise and worship. I ceased to dread my visits to the loo since they became extraordinarily profitable occasions.

Slowly I tried to exercise my body. It was an exceptionally cold time of the year, but protected with coat, scarf and hat I ventured a few yards along the street, only to hobble straight back for another lengthy session in my customary sitting-down position. Soon I was walking a little further, and every day I tried to extend those walks as far as I possibly could, setting myself specific targets each day.

For two lovely weeks I went to a farm in Sussex at the invitation of great personal friends, Michael and Gillie Warren, and each walk in the wintry Sussex countryside became times of special communion with God. In certain directions the piercing wind stung my face, but on the way home I felt its force almost pushing me up the gentle hill. I prayed that I might know the direction of the wind of the Spirit for my future ministry, and kept on asking, 'Lord what do you want me to do?'

I noticed the first green shoots miraculously pushing their way through the hard, cold soil; and I thanked God that the life of his Spirit could also overcome the toughest barriers, including those cancer cells. Even the bare trees bore the promise of life. 'If Winter comes, can Spring be far behind?' As I walked I worshipped him, talked to him, listened to him, and thoroughly enjoyed his presence in the midst of his creation.

Anne herself, however, was now far from well. In less than

a week after my return from hospital she was in bed all day
with pains in her kidneys, pains from a stomach ulcer and a
palpitating heart. These troubles continued for many weeks,
and although she went to the doctor several times for various
tests, it became increasingly clear that these were purely
symptoms of stress. It was not surprising. Anne had experienced considerable stress during our last year or two in York;
this was followed by a most painful time when we moved to
London, since for months we felt almost bereaved having lost
our church family with whom we had been for seventeen
years; and then of course she suffered substantial strains
through my illness and prognosis. During the immediate
crisis in hospital, Anne was an absolute tower of strength.
Now that I was home again, the tensions began to emerge in
her body. It was not an easy time.

   Added to that, various people began to send us endless
books and articles on cures for cancer. Every one of them was
a thoughtful and generous gesture, but together they brought
us (Anne in particular) under colossal pressure. Most of the
publications gave the impression that providing we followed
a certain line of treatment precisely, there was just a possibility that I might be healed. Many of the books suggested
special diets, and these often differed from one another,
which we found most confusing; and together they gave Anne
the gut-feeling that my life was in her hands. If she bought
the right food, and prepared it in the right way, and kept me
on the right treatment, all might be well; but if she failed to do
this, the future was bleak. As I saw her becoming more and
more tense with each new book arriving, I realised that any
marginal benefit emerging from a better diet would be
cancelled out immediately by the marked increase of tensions
in our lives and relationship. Although I do not doubt that
some people can benefit from a strict diet and perhaps even
overcome cancer in this way, we felt that simple adjustments,
such as an increase of fruit and raw vegetables and a general
avoidance of unnecessary toxins, was all that we could
handle peacefully.

Nine days after my return home, I had to go to the hospital as an outpatient for my first ultra-sound scan. Everything seemed to go wrong. To begin with our boiler backfired that morning, emitting nauseating fumes throughout the house, and all the central heating was off for a week. It was February and distinctly cold. I nearly fainted in the shower, partly from the fumes, and partly because I wasn't allowed any food before a scan.

When we arrived at the ultra-sound unit, I was told to remove my clothes and put on a paper gown together with a small, thin, ill-fitting cotton robe. I felt semi-naked, and we had to sit in a freezing corridor (I was chilled to the bone) for no less than an hour and a half. It was only three weeks after my operation, and I was feeling far from well. Perhaps these factors coloured my impressions, but for me the whole setting looked bleak. The corridor in which we sat was totally bare without even colourful posters to relieve the institutional painted walls; other very sick cancer patients were waiting their turn with an air of hopeless resignation; and the scan itself seemed not only an assessment of cancer, but a doom-watch of life itself. It reminded me of Solzhenitsyn's *Cancer Ward*, a brilliant but despairing book. The combination of factors surrounding my visit were utterly depressing, clinical, negative and entirely devoid of hope. My spirits, which had been largely on top until now, sank to a record low, and it was several days before I began to recover. Although I am sure that this was far from the hospital's intention, I *felt* little more than a slab of meat placed before sophisticated scientific instruments for the benefit of measuring disease. I was no longer a person with human emotions, fears and forebodings, struggling to maintain some positive hope.

In contrast to this the attitude of Dr Harper, my specialist in the Medical Oncology Clinic whom I saw five weeks later, was marvellous. His thoroughly positive and personal approach, seeing both Anne and me together and discussing all sorts of details of our life, helped to restore confidence. His small clinic was full of attractive posters and served by a cheerful staff.

Nevertheless I have to say that I found most of my visits as an outpatient undoubtedly depressing. Nearly always there have been long and, even worse, unexplained delays. No one knows why nothing *seems* to be happening. On one occasion I sat for an hour and a half on a tiny chair designed for a very small child (there was no alternative), only to be told at last that I was in the wrong queue for an X-ray, even though I had been expressly sent to that area.

On another occasion I was sent by my specialist to the same X-ray unit to book an appointment for another ultra-sound scan. After the usual delays, I was told to go to a certain waiting area for an X-ray. I protested, insisting that I should have a scan, not an X-ray. I was overruled, however, and made to go for an X-ray. After I had waited for the rest of the afternoon, a nurse came to say that I was sitting in the wrong place since I needed a scan! These are only trivial points, but the accumulation of inefficiency, of being pushed here and there, of unexplained delays, combined with the impersonality of the whole procedure, created an entirely negative atmosphere which must surely hinder the healing process. At a later date, and with the full agreement of my own doctor, I signed myself off as an outpatient.

For some time I knew the powerful effect that positive and negative influences could have on our health. John Wimber gave me the details of a fascinating book called *Anatomy Of An Illness*, by Norman Cousins.[1] In this book the author describes his own remarkable healing from ankylosing spondy-litis, which means the disintegration of the connective tissues in the spine. One specialist gave him only one chance in five hundred for full recovery, although that specialist admitted that he had personally never seen anyone recover from that condition. Cousins found it increasingly difficult moving his limbs, his jaws were almost locked and nodules appeared on his body.

[1] Published by Bantam Books, 1981.

Years before, Cousins had read Hans Selye's famous book *The Stress of Life*, where the author describes the damaging effects of negative emotions on body chemistry. 'The inevitable question arose in my mind,' commented Cousins, 'what about the positive emotions? If negative emotions produce negative chemical changes in the body, wouldn't the positive emotions produce positive chemical changes? Is it possible that love, hope, faith, laughter, confidence, and the will to live have therapeutic value? Do chemical changes occur only on the downside?'

There was no doubt concerning Cousins' determination to live, despite the medical prognosis, and together with his doctor (who was wholly supportive), he planned a radical treatment for his disease. To begin with, he obtained a lot of comedy films, such as *Candid Camera* and the old Marx Brothers classics. 'We pulled down the blinds and turned on the machine. It worked. I made the joyous discovery that ten minutes of genuine belly laughter had an anaesthetic effect and would give me at least two hours of pain-free sleep.' His blood sedimentation rate readings also dropped consistently after each episode of laughter. He removed himself out of hospital as soon as he could, and went to a hotel room instead which he found much more pleasant and costing only a third of the price (there is no National Health Service in America). With the approval of his doctor, Cousins also prescribed for himself massive doses of vitamin C. Immediately the sedimentation rate dropped significantly further. 'Seldom had I known such elation. The ascorbic acid was working. So was laughter. The combination was cutting heavily into whatever poison was attacking the connective tissue.'

Before long he was completely off drugs and sleeping well. The recovery took many months, and even now is not entirely complete. But for years Cousins has been able to lead a full life, playing tennis and golf, riding horses and playing Bach's *Toccata and Fugue in D Minor* (one of his specific ambitions). The full details of the story are intriguing.

What is particularly important, and this is a point readily

backed by most doctors, is that no medication available is as potent as the state of mind that a patient brings to his or her own illness. It seems now incontrovertible that chemical changes in the body do take place as a result of mental attitudes or moods. 'The brain produces encephalins and endorphins, which moderate pain and help set a stage for recovery. The brain plays a part in the production of gamma globulin, which is vital for the body's immune system. The brain produces interferon, which acts as a cancer-blocking agent. The vast array of substances produced by the brain are all connected to human development, to the fulfilment of human potentialities, to the maintenance of health, and to the war against disease. What is more significant about this process is that the brain's secretions can be stimulated or diminished by thought and behaviour and environment.'[2] Our thoughts, attitudes and reactions to all the many facets surrounding a serious illness are of paramount importance in the process of recovery.

[2]*Human Options* by Norman Cousins, Berkley Books, New York, 1983.

13

Strength out of Weakness

Well-meaning visitors can be a problem for anyone who is trying slowly to recuperate. We had endless letters and telephone calls from friends and acquaintances who wanted to see me, talk to me, pray with me and in various ways encourage me. Anne and Hilary were polite but ruthless! At the most they allowed only one visitor a day for the first few weeks, and even those were screened carefully. Some people are always refreshing, but others, with the best of intentions, can be exhausting.

Our first and a very welcome guest was the television personality and cookery expert, Delia Smith, who had written one or two extremely helpful letters when I was in hospital and who had sent a superb arrangement of flowers. Both Anne and I had become very fond of Delia in the comparatively short time since we had known her. Delia invariably brings with her a delightful breath of fresh life and joy, springing from her own deepening relationship with Christ. We loved having her in our home.

'You have been an activist like Simon Peter,' said Delia to me. 'I believe that Jesus now wants you to be more like the apostle John, calling you closer to him and teaching you to listen to him. There will be a new quality in your ministry as a result.'

I listened carefully, willing for God to do whatever he liked in my life. Delia also shared a prophetic word about me given through a close personal friend of hers, Frances Hogan:

The Lord is staking his claim on you. There comes a point in the spiritual life when your apostolate is not more important than your relationship with the Lord. He becomes very jealous of your relationship with him. He has done what the shepherd sometimes does to the sheep. He is not beyond breaking the leg of the sheep in order to save its life. He then heals the leg by binding it up and puts the sheep on his shoulder until it learns a new stage of intimacy with him.

Apparently Frances had also said,

I don't feel the cancer will kill, if you make this deep surrender to the Lord. The Lord wants to bring you to complete identification with Christ's suffering as well as his glory. This is to bring you to the stage of 'I do only what my Father tells me to do, and I say only what my Father tells me to say'. To reach this stage there must be a deeper prayer life – and you must let go some of the apostolate.

As I listened to Delia, I felt that the Lord was speaking directly to me.

My response was to repent of the busyness that had all too often squeezed out any real depth of prayer. Once again I surrendered everything I could think of to the Lord: my work, my travelling, my team, my future, my family and even my life. Every day I sought to renew this surrender, telling God that I was happy with him alone and with whatever he chose to give me. I wanted to take my hands off the reins so that God could do what he wanted in my life. And I would continue to praise him. I thought again of those words from Psalm 16:

> You, Lord, are all I have,
> and you give me all I need;
> my future is in your hands . . .

I found great peace. When we surrender everything to God, we can never lose. It is only when we try to grasp some things for ourselves that one day we shall forfeit them. I remembered those words of Jesus: 'For whoever would save his life will lose it; and whoever loses his life for my sake and the gospel's will save it' (Mark 8:35). I began to discover a new quality of life and my relationship with Jesus seemed to have more depth.

A few days later we were especially glad to welcome Bishop Morris and Anne Maddocks. Morris had been the Bishop of Selby for ten years during our time in York, and we always had the closest relationship with both of them. We loved them, respected them, and often benefited from their wise and gracious healing ministry. This time they came for the express purpose of holding a Communion Service (a 'Eucharist of the Resurrection' as Morris called it) in our home.

There are few more warm and encouraging couples than Morris and Anne. We were thrilled that they could come, and their emphasis on both word and sacrament was one that we appreciated. We covered a table in our drawing-room with a white cloth, and put two candles on it, each ringed with small flowers at their base. It was an unusual but attractive communion table.

Morris put on his bishop's purple cassock and white rochet, and we turned to the collect and readings set for the eighth Sunday before Easter, in the *Alternative Service Book*. They could not have been more appropriate if we had carefully chosen them ourselves:

Almighty and everliving God
whose Son Jesus Christ healed the sick
and restored them to wholeness of life:
look with compassion on the anguish of the world,
and by your healing power
make whole both men and nations . . .

The Old Testament reading was from Zephaniah 3: '. . . The Lord is in your midst; you shall fear evil no more . . . I will remove disaster from you . . .'

Then came a reading from James 5:

Is any among you sick? Let him call for the elders of the church, and let them pray over him, anointing him with oil in the name of the Lord; and the prayer of faith will save the sick man, and the Lord will raise him up . . .

The Gospel too was about the healing of the paralysed man. In fact the whole emphasis was on God's power to heal and save. We read the passages and spent a few moments meditating on their relevance, with Morris guiding our thoughts.

Guy unfortunately was away at school, but Anne, Fiona and I, together with Morris and Anne, were deeply aware of the Lord's presence in that room. We received the tokens of God's forgiveness and love, and at the appropriate moment Morris anointed me with oil, laying hands upon me and praying for me. It was a time of deep peace and much personal blessing. In many ways it was totally different from the style of John Wimber and his two friends; and yet both forms of ministries, however different, seemed to bring the healing power of God into our lives.

Morris and Anne stayed for a quick tea, as we talked and laughed together. However they had a long journey ahead of them and were already late, so reluctantly we let them go. Our whole house seemed full of God's peace for the rest of that weekend. I knew that my life was safely in God's hands.

The next week, when I was recuperating on their farm in Sussex, Michael and Gillie Warren protected me almost totally from visitors. But I was especially glad to make two exceptions. The first was a visit from the American leaders of my team, Mark and Carol Slomka, who had just returned from their five weeks in California. I knew they had all been praying and fasting for me, and I treasured the letters that I had received from them in the midst of their hectic programme. When I saw Mark and Carol I gave each of them a long hug. It was so wonderful seeing them again. I realised how closely God had brought us together as a team, and how our relationships had deepened through my illness and enforced absence. It was marvellous hearing all the news of how everything had gone in California without me. As usual, I found out that I was quite dispensable! However, I could not wait to see the rest of the team as well.

The next day I had a lightning visit from an outstanding Christian leader in South Africa, Michael Cassidy, and his sister Olave Snelling. Michael and I have been together only for brief meetings over the years, but he once graciously introduced me at a ministers' meeting in Vancouver (where he happened to be at the time) by saying, 'I know of no other Christian leader in the world with whom I identify so completely, and with whom I share my vision so fully.' I was tremendously moved by those words, and Michael and I have always felt 'of one heart and mind' as brothers in Christ.

'We love you deeply,' said Michael, 'and thousands of black Christians and white Christians are praying for your complete healing.'

After a quick lunch, we stood together in a circle and prayed for one another. Then Michael and Olave sped away, trying to reach Heathrow in time to catch Michael's plane to Johannesburg. It was only a short visit, but immensely encouraging. Michael urged me to catch the 'thermal of the Spirit' – to see what God was doing and to go in his direction, strengthened by his power.

Monday, March 7th was my fiftieth birthday! Some of my friends who had reached that milestone before me had enjoyed all sorts of unusual and intriguing celebrations. Mine passed by almost unnoticed, except for some cards and presents mostly from my family. But then I was not up to anything else. However, the doorbell rang in the middle of the morning and there was my team singing on my doorstep and presenting me with a huge birthday card. It was the first time I had seen them all since my operation, and we had a

great hour together. It had not been easy for them going to
California without me and having to work with two speakers
they had never met before. But undoubtedly they had grown
spiritually more mature as a result. In particular they had
experienced a fresh spiritual renewal with John Wimber and
members of his church, which had given them a new vision of
God and of the work of his Spirit.

I had promised my Trustees and surgeon that I would do
no work until Easter at the earliest. Much of my day was
spent in my small book-lined study, reading the Bible and
praying, going through the various services in the ASB (the
modern Anglican Prayer Book) and listening to numerous
cassettes, mostly in the loo. Sometimes I would keep my
recorder in the loo all ready! It was a relaxed time, reading,
listening, walking, eating and sleeping.

When I was asked, however, by Chris Rees of the BBC if I
would do a radio interview with Nick Page, I felt strongly
that I ought to agree. It was only two months after my
operation and I was still far from strong, tiring easily after
any mental or physical exertion, but the BBC team came
round to my home for the recording. Nick Page asked some
excellent questions, and I answered as best I could about my
personal feelings and experiences over the past two months
in particular.

I always enjoy such interviews, partly because in a natural
and relaxed way I can talk about Christ and about the
tremendous quality of life he brings to us, not least a glorious
hope for the future – a hope based solidly on his own resurrection.

'But what happens,' asked Nick Page, 'if you find that
healing is not coming?'

'If I found it was not coming, I hope I have got to the
position of really trusting in Christ that the best is yet to be.
You know, actually to be with Christ and free for ever from
the pain and suffering, tears and all the problems and
injustices of this world, there is nothing more glorious than
that. That is why I genuinely am at the place where I really

want to be in heaven (sometimes the sooner the better), but I am willing to be on this earth, with all its struggles and battles if he wants me here.'

The interview lasted for an hour, and it stimulated me instead of exhausting me. Chris and Nick seemed pleased, but I had no idea of the interest the edited half-hour programme would cause. It was called *David Watson – A Case for Healing?* and we were deluged with correspondence in response to the broadcast. I have a PO Box, and poor Hilary or Anne would stagger back day after day with bags full of letters. Over a thousand were received within a few weeks. I wrote a general newsletter giving some basic information and expressing my appreciation for the enormous concern and prayer I was receiving from so many different places, so that Hilary was able to answer nearly all the letters received, mostly with the newsletter. Some letters were cries for help. Hilary did what she could, but obviously we could not say very much.

The programme was so well received that it was repeated on Radio 4 five weeks later, and subsequently on the World Service of the BBC. I heard of several people driving home from work who pulled into the side of the road to listen carefully to it. One gifted young doctor, who described himself as a militant atheist, heard the programme, was deeply moved by it, and that same evening read a book I had written which one of his partners had given him a year before. Totally against his normal self-contained personality, he burst into tears and, feeling rather foolish, knelt down to ask Christ into his life. His conversion was remarkable, and a few weeks later his startled wife also thoughtfully committed her life to Christ.

The BBC had taken the precautionary measure of having the recorded cassette of the broadcast available for sale.[1] Many hundreds were sold, with probably thousands more

[1] Cassette available from Anchor Recordings, 72 The Street, Kennington, Ashford, Kent, TN24 9HS.

privately recorded or re-recorded! Careful not to make too
many enquiries about this, I was staggered by the number of
people in many parts of the world who heard the broadcast,
and equally amazed by the impact it was apparently making.
It was a reminder to me of the enormous interest in (or
anxiety about?) death. It is our one future certainty, and
there are no answers to it – apart from Christ.

I was aware of the danger of being given undue publicity
because of my open fight against cancer, but I was concerned
to talk freely about that 'dreaded disease'. The only way to
conquer fears is to face them. Added to that, I wanted to
share the wonderful hope that we have as Christians, whatever the future may hold, and to speak honestly about my
experiences of God's love and power in the midst of human
struggles and anxieties. We had to refuse several journalists
wanting interviews, following the broadcast, but I gave my
time and energy to as many as I could manage.

Michael Green, the Rector of St Aldate's Church in
Oxford and for many years a close personal friend, was kind
enough to suggest that the radio interview might emerge as
the most powerful and influential talk I had ever given! And
yet all I did was to sit in my armchair, still very weak, trying
to answer the questions that Nick Page put to me. If God had
used that interview to touch the lives of people in many parts
of the world, it was (for me) another indication that Christ's
power is most effective in our weakness.

14

Planning for a Future

'Where shall we go?' I asked.

Maps and brochures were spread before us, with Anne, Fiona and Guy breaking in with various suggestions.

'How about Polzeath in Cornwall? Or the Lake District?'

'If we want the sun at Easter, why not Florida?' said Guy hopefully.

We had been given by a number of friends generous sums of money for recuperation, and for once in our lifetime we agreed that we would go as a family to a hotel. Always before we had borrowed cottages from our friends. In fact, Anne and I had never stayed in a hotel since our honeymoon nineteen years before (when I was seriously ill with asthma), so that our children had never known such a luxury. It had been far too expensive and out of the question.

This time would be a special occasion. Anne had been far from well over the weeks, and even by Easter she was still suffering from a spastic colon and palpitations in her heart; so I was anxious that she should not have to shop, cook and clean. Fiona and Guy had also suffered from the tensions of the past months. So we were going to spoil ourselves – for a whole week!

After poring over books, hotel guides and maps, we eventually settled on a hotel we had never heard of, in Devon, and found to our delight that they had room for us for the week we had chosen.

Highbullen Hotel, Chittlehamholt in North Devon, was as delightful as its name suggests. Set in a beautiful estate,

complete with its own herd of deer, it had about it the
atmosphere of a peaceful country club. Anxious to have a
quiet week, we had deliberately chosen a hotel where children under thirteen were not allowed, and we were free to
enjoy the privacy of our own family life or mingle with a few
guests, whichever we preferred. The food was outstanding
and the rooms were comfortable. Most important of all,
especially for Guy, there were wonderful facilities available.
Every morning before breakfast Guy went for a swim in the
indoor swimming pool (even I went in once or twice!). Then
after breakfast it was a constant round of activities. Each day
Guy and I played tennis, squash, golf and snooker (all on the
premises) – Anne and Fiona joining in as they wished. I
don't think I can remember a holiday when I had been so
energetic, and this was only three months after my major
operation! Most important of all, it was *quality* time for us
together as a family. We knew that we might never have such
a holiday again, at least because of the expense, but we
enjoyed every minute of it and felt incredibly refreshed by it.

The Devon countryside was magnificent in spring, with
myriads of primroses bursting forth everywhere, especially in
the banks of the narrow country lanes. It was the time of year
when life was rising out of death, fresh beauty peeping round
every corner with unexpected glory. Newborn lambs were
skipping with joy, and the whole atmosphere breathed hope.
It was good to be alive.

Guy and I also had a good long talk about my illness as we
walked together one afternoon. 'Gosh!' he said, 'I had no idea
that it was so serious. I'm glad you didn't tell me too much
when I was away at school last term.' In fact I was amazed by
the calm way in which he took it all, asking intelligent
questions about the operation, about what a colostomy
would have meant, and about the future. He was simply
marvellous: free, frank, honest, uninhibited – just Guy. I was
proud to be his father.

Naturally I talked to Fiona too from time to time. And in
spite of the constant tensions surrounding her at home (with

inevitable visits to the hospital, results from scans, etc), she was normally her steady unruffled self and often full of fun. I found her constantly supportive and remarkably caring when she could see I was tired.

We returned home just in time for the children to start their new term at school; and then Anne and I flew out to California to spend ten days with John and Carol Wimber, attending their church services on two Sundays. It was Anne's first visit there, and a few weeks previously she was not at all sure that she wanted to go. Anne always finds it difficult meeting lots of new people (perhaps especially so if I know them already), and she was also anxious about my state of health and about her own pains and palpitations. However we went.

The flight was not too difficult for me at all, although we were glad to arrive at Los Angeles, at about three a.m. by British time. John and Carol were away for a couple of days, but we had a marvellous welcome from Bob and Penny Fulton, whom I had come to love dearly over the last four years. Bob is the assistant-pastor with John Wimber. Thoughtfully and generously they took us to a comfortable motel for two nights, to help us recover from the flight before moving to John and Carol's home. I saw Anne relax as soon as Bob and Penny met us. I knew she would, because I had so often experienced their open, loving and accepting friendship where there is no need to say the right words or do the right things before you are welcomed. I knew that they, and others in their church, loved people unconditionally – and it is a love which quickly drives away all fears and melts down all barriers.

At our first service in that church on Sunday morning I noticed Anne shaking a little before the service had even started. Was she nervous or cold?

'I just *knew* that God was with us,' she explained afterwards. 'I somehow felt the power of God in my body and I couldn't help shaking!'

I never seem to feel anything on these occasions, but I

loved being there: the warmth and love of the congregation, the reality and intimacy of sustained worship, the sense of quiet expectation throughout, and excellent biblical teaching. God was undoubtedly present, whether anyone shook or not!

Before the evening service started, I asked John Wimber if I might say a few words to thank everyone for praying for me.

'Sure,' he replied. 'They'd like that.'

So at an appropriate spot in the service John announced that Anne and I were present and that I wanted to say a few words.

I was totally unprepared for what followed. As soon as I stood up, everyone (over 3,000 of them) clapped and clapped and clapped. They even stood and went on clapping and clapping. It was like a standing ovation. I would have been terribly embarrassed, except for two things. In the first place I knew that this was a spontaneous expression of their love, and I was not embarrassed by their love – just deeply moved by it. I also knew that this was a 'clap-offering' to the Lord – a way of saying 'thank you' to God for visibly answering their prayers for my healing. It suddenly struck me how much they must have prayed and fasted for me, since they exploded with such applause when I stood up. It was an unforgettable experience.

'Those guys really love you,' said John afterwards.

'I don't know why, but I guess they do,' I replied, still not quite able to take it all in.

During that weekend we kept on meeting people who had been healed from all sorts of complaints and diseases, from backaches to cancer. No wonder nearly a hundred streamed through after the evening service for prayer and counselling. Some asked for healing, some wanted to find Christ, some longed to be filled with the Spirit. But in quiet, relaxed and unemotional ways many from the congregation (some quite young) were praying with those who were needing help. God was manifestly at work amongst them all.

Much of our time with John and Carol that week was spent

in laughter! I don't think Anne and I have laughed so much for years, and it was a refreshing change from the unhealthy intensity of some Christian groups we know. Of course that church also knew when to be serious, when to pray, when to praise, and when to be still before God. They were anything but superficial and flippant. But they had discovered some of the abundant quality of life that Jesus comes to bring, and had learnt how to enjoy all that was good.

We also had some excellent discussions and times of prayer together. John called in some of the 'kids' to pray for us – young people mostly between the ages of eighteen and twenty-three – and we were impressed by the quality of their relationships with God and with one another. They were spiritually alive, sensitive to the Holy Spirit, and full of faith. Admittedly they were not yet fully mature in Christ. Most of them had been Christians for only two or three years. But their loving and prayerful ministry towards us was astonishing.

We had one more marvellous Sunday with them all, and then we flew home. There is nothing in the world like being consciously in God's presence, surrounded by the love of his people. It is literally a foretaste of heaven. I have known many happy experiences during my lifetime, but nothing can be compared to the caring love, wholesome joy and prevailing peace that only God can bring. 'Your presence fills me with joy and brings me pleasure for ever' (Psalm 16:11, *Good News Bible*).

As we approached London Anne's pains and palpitations, which had vanished in California, suddenly returned. Also within a few days I had another scan on my liver which revealed that the cancer was still increasing. As I spoke to John Wimber on the phone, I knew he was stunned by the news.

'We really believe that God *is* healing you,' said John. 'With cancer, it sometimes gets worse before it begins to die. We'll go on praying, and if necessary we'll come straight over and pray with you some more.'

'Thanks John. I'll keep in touch.' At least I was feeling fit and ready for work again.

At this stage I was thinking and praying constantly about my future work, especially since it affected my team of eight who were now not as busy as they would have been if I had not been off work. Under the leadership of Bob Roxburgh they were marvellously fulfilling the engagements I had accepted months previously, but what was God saying to us about our long-term future?

I found it confusing. In some ways I find guidance, if anything, gets harder rather than easier the longer I am a Christian. Perhaps God allows this so that we have to go on relying on him and not on ourselves.

To begin with, I thought that we should try to buy a redundant theatre in the centre of London, to try to com-municate the Christian Gospel in ways that many have found meaningful, even when they had been disillusioned by the Church. Certainly I could use the creative gifts of the team to full advantage in such a setting. It became obvious, however, that a venture of this nature would prove enormously expen-sive, and it was too early to expect people to give money for a work that hinged largely upon a man who was supposedly dying of cancer!

Next I considered taking over one or two of the churches in central London that were all but redundant. The Bishop of London was enthusiastic about my proposals, but as Anne and I went round many possible churches our hearts sank. The buildings were all unsuitable: too small, too badly in need of repair or too depressing for our purposes. We were offered one church with considerable potential, but I said to the Bishop, 'If I were forty and fit I would jump at it, but now that I'm fifty and frail I honestly think it is too much.' He agreed.

My team had to be very patient. Now that I was meeting regularly with them, I was coming up with a new suggestion about our future almost every week – only to find it frus-trated a little later. If cancer was one problem I battled with, confusion was certainly another. Yet, if it seemed right for me to spend more time in London and less time travelling, I wanted to get my teeth into something that was both challenging and demanding. My Trustees also had to be patient, since at every meeting they had to consider a new proposal from me. Although I kept praying about the future, I still could not see clearly the way ahead. I felt like a tourist in London, standing in the middle of Hyde Park Corner in thick fog. Several voices were calling me in different directions, but I still could not hear the Lord.

Added to that, the Trustees had a responsibility towards the various committees that had invited me (or were thinking of doing so) for certain events in the future. What plans could we realistically make when medically-speaking the prognosis was so poor? How far would committees be willing to plan a festival in eighteen months' time, involving a fair amount of time and money, when there was no guarantee that I would be there to lead it? The Trustees felt it right to send out a letter in June explaining the position as honestly and as accurately as possible:

We invite the persistent prayers of the Church at large for complete healing. David's present vigour and his increasing appetite for work are consistent with the view that healing is taking place and that his specialist's prescription for an active and long-term ministry is right.

We believe that an inevitable change in policy must be accepted after this illness. The gruelling international programme which involved so much travelling must be curtailed to some extent and a more settled ministry in London should be developed. The trustees were coming to this opinion before the illness, which has dramatically confirmed it. David is perhaps one of the most gifted communicators of the Christian faith and widely accepted across all boundaries in this land as well as elsewhere. We are making plans for his gifts to be used in London on a regular basis, with a special emphasis on training Chris-

tians to develop their own gifts of ministry for the benefit of
others. Details of what precisely this will mean are not yet
available, but the general concept reveals our faith in
God's purposes for David in the future.

The travelling ministry of inter-church festivals and
missions, and also training programmes in seminaries and
for ministers, will continue. It is plain, however, that those
responsible for initiating these events at the local level must
be able to share in our faith and join in our prayers for
healing to continue. We do not expect for some time to be
able to offer further medical evidence which would lift the
responsibility off local committees to make their decisions
in the light of the present facts, and therefore we are
content to accept only such invitations for David as are
made with the present medical condition fully understood.
We are convinced that our own 'risk' of faith is both
reasonable and responsible, but we must ask those who
invite David to accept their responsibility to decide in
faith. It is important that they should be at peace about
their decision.

It was a clear letter, but I was not altogether surprised when
one Christian leader, responsible for a major event overseas
involving the whole team, telephoned me to ask if I would be
well in a year's time! How was I to reply to that? James wrote
in his New Testament letter: 'How do you know what is going
to happen tomorrow? For the length of your lives is as
uncertain as the morning fog – now you see it; soon it is gone.
What you ought to say is, "If the Lord wants us to, we shall
live and do this or that" ' (4:13–16, *Living Bible*). In all our
plans about the future we are entirely dependent upon the
Lord who both gives life, and takes it away.

Never before had I been so uncertain about life and work.
At times I was so confused about the future that I wondered if
there could be any future at all for me on this earth. It was a
tense and anxious stage in my life. I was tempted to question
repeatedly the decision to leave York. In some ways every-

thing would have been much easier had we stayed there.

During this period of convalescence I had time to reflect on a number of basic priorities. Both Anne and I had been exhausted after seventeen exciting but demanding years in York, and spiritually, mentally, emotionally and physically we were nearly 'burnt out'. The Archbishop of York had advised us to have a sabbatical leave a few years previously, but with our children at school it seemed impossible. Unexpectedly we were now having our sabbatical rest, not in the way we imagined, but we were more refreshed and more together as a family than we had been for a long time.

15

A Fifth Dimension

'This is a day of decision,' said Dr Harper, my specialist, when I saw him in May. 'I'm afraid that the scan shows a considerable increase of the cancer in the liver.'

I was a little stunned since I hadn't expected that. I was now feeling remarkably well, physically more active than I had been for some time, and it would not have surprised me if the cancer had already disappeared. I said nothing.

'I think we must put you on to some chemotherapy,' said Dr Harper.

'I'm sorry,' I replied, 'but I definitely don't want that.'

'Are you sure?'

'Quite sure.'

'You've thought out your decision carefully?'

'Yes,' I replied, though I was glad that he did not press me for my reasons there and then. The consultation ended rather abruptly, and Anne and I returned home considerably subdued.

Several people had reminded us of the incident in the Gospels about the fig-tree as a parable of what might be happening. The tree did not die when Jesus cursed it; it withered only later. Perhaps this was what the tumour in my liver was doing, suggested Anne.

Perhaps. With a terminal illness I felt as though I were walking on a tight-rope of faith. It required only the smallest knock to make me feel very insecure. Perhaps no healing was happening after all. Perhaps the disease was taking its usual course. I was undoubtedly depressed, and I feared the worst.

During the next week or two my decision to refuse chemotherapy was tested several times, although Anne shared my decision completely. Several doctors, including some close friends, gently urged me to think again. At the same time I was making my own enquiries. When I asked a few doctors and specialists to be totally honest with me, nearly all admitted that chemotherapy did not heal cancer in the liver. At best the patient's life might be extended a little, but the quality of life could suffer considerably through the effects of the treatment. As time went on, a growing number of the medical profession told me that they felt I had made the right decision.

Added to the dubious results of chemotherapy on cancer of the liver (I understand it can be much more successful with other types of cancer), I was determined to avoid as much negative influence as I possibly could, and I did not want to spend my remaining days (however many or few) waiting in the Outpatients Department of Guy's Hospital.

Moreover, as I listened to numerous teaching cassettes on healing – mostly by John Wimber – and as I studied my New Testament more thoroughly, I became fascinated by the 'fifth dimension' that Christ introduced when he both proclaimed and demonstrated the Kingdom of God.

We live today in a hostile and fractured world. Everywhere we find a profound sense of alienation. We are alienated from God, hence the spiritual confusion and unreality that many experience. We are alienated from one another, hence broken marriages, violence on the streets and hostility between nations. We are alienated from the environment, hence the ravages of hunger, poverty, disease and pollution. We are also alienated from ourselves, hence the mental and psychological afflictions which cause distress in our lives.

It was into such an alienation that Jesus came nearly 2,000 years ago. He saw people as 'harassed and helpless' – a poignantly accurate description of our society today. What is the answer to the tangle of human suffering that ensnares us all, one way or another? It is not education, since tragically the staggering technological progress made in the last few decades now threatens to destroy us all. Nor is it politics. New policies may change the structures of a nation, but until the heart of man is renewed nothing will be significantly different.

Jesus came as the Great Restorer, the Healer of broken lives and relationships. He began his brief but astonishing ministry by saying, 'The time is fulfilled, and the kingdom of God is at hand; repent and believe in the Gospel' (Mark 1:15). Frequently he taught about the kingdom: there are one hundred references to the kingdom in the first three Gospels alone. He gave instructions about entering the kingdom, he urged his disciples to pray for the coming of the kingdom, he illustrated the kingdom in parables and spoke about the future blessings of the kingdom. He also demonstrated the power of the kingdom.

What, then, is the kingdom? In the Bible it means specifically the *authority and rule of a king*. So the kingdom of God means the rule or reign of God. When Jesus came preaching the kingdom he was introducing God's New Society: a new age had come. There was now release for those who were captive to the old order of sin, suffering and death. It was not that those enemies of man were now banished. But those who sinned could be forgiven, those who were sick could be healed, and those who died in Christ would be more alive than ever.

One of the most helpful definitions of the kingdom is that given by Hans Küng: 'God's kingdom is creation healed.' Saviour means healer. Salvation is much wider than the forgiveness of sins (all-important as that is); it means *wholeness*, with God's authority and rule affecting every area of our lives. Christ has come to bring peace on earth and so end the alienation which sooner or later destroys us all.

For many years I had been convinced that, through Christ and through his death on the cross, our relationships with God and with one another could be healed. What fascinated me afresh was the space given in the Gospel records to the healing ministry of Christ – a ministry which continued by the power of the Holy Spirit through the disciples in the early Church.

It was clear that Jesus healed *all* who came to him. He never turned anyone away. A leper once came to him and said, 'Lord, if you will, you can make me clean.' At once Jesus stretched out his hand to touch him and said, 'I will; be clean' (Matthew 8:1–3). It is unthinkable that Jesus could have replied, 'Sorry, but this leprosy is for the good of your soul!'

At the same time I noticed that there was a mystery about the healings of Jesus. In the Pool of Bethesda there was 'a multitude' of sick people. Jesus stepped across them and healed only one. Why? I don't know. When the Centurion's servant was sick, Jesus healed him from a distance; he did not have to be there. Why could he not do this with all the sick in Palestine at that time? I don't know.

The difficulty may be all part of the 'now' and 'not yet' of the Kingdom of God. The Kingdom has now come, since Christ has come to be our Saviour and King; but it will not yet be consummated until Christ comes again with power and glory. Even where healings are experienced widely not all sick people are healed. Christ taught us to pray 'Your Kingdom come', and we are still to wait with patience for what we see only in part at present.

Because of the 'not yet' of the Kingdom, I could not accept the more extreme view contained in quite a few letters: 'Once you have claimed God's healing, you've got it!' I knew this was based on the general promise of Jesus: 'Whatever you ask in prayer, believe that you have received it, and it will be yours' (Mark 11:24). But some texts read, '. . . believe that you *are receiving it* . . .' This I could accept. Over the months I have often said publicly, 'I believe that God is in the process of healing me. Every day I thank him that he is healing me. But, logically speaking, it is possible that I am wrong.' God only knows.

I saw too that Jesus healed out of compassion. This was the motivation that prompted Jesus to spend himself for the

poor, the sick and the needy. There is great healing power in
love, especially the love of God. What helped me more than
anything was the expression of that love through numerous
Christians who obviously cared for me, prayed for me,
encouraged me, thus surrounding me with the love of God.

Jesus also healed when there was a prevailing atmosphere
of faith. Four men once brought a paralysed friend to Jesus,
and they were so determined that they broke up the roof of a
house and lowered their friend to the feet of Jesus since there
was no other possible way of getting through the crowds.
That took some initiative. When Jesus saw *their* faith, he
forgave the sick man his sins and healed him of his paralysis.
Clearly this unusual demonstration of faith helped towards
the miracle of healing.

On the other hand, even Jesus was hindered by unbelief.
At his own home town, Nazareth, he could do 'no mighty
work . . . because of their unbelief'. He could heal only a few
sick people (Mark 6:5f). I have found that my own faith in
God's healing is inevitably vulnerable, and influenced to
some extent by the faith or unbelief of those around me.
Constantly I need to encourage my faith by worshipping God
and by reading his word; but on top of that, the supportive-
believing prayer of others, especially my team, has been a
vital factor in the 'fight of faith' over these past months.

Jesus also healed more effectively when the Spirit of God
was moving in power. 'The power of the Lord was with him
to heal' (Luke 5:17). I am not quite sure what this means,
since Jesus was constantly full of the Spirit of God. But I
thought of that first day when John Wimber and the two
others came to see me. They had not expected to spend time
praying with me then, but they became aware of 'the power
of the Lord' coming upon them. I have also known times
when healings *flow*, one after another, without any apparent
effort in terms of prayer, counselling or whatever – simply
because the power of God is unusually present.

Jesus sometimes had to pray more than once. After he
prayed for a blind man, he asked, 'Do you see anything?' The

man replied, 'I see men; but they look like trees, walking.' So Jesus laid hands on his eyes again, and this time sight was fully restored (Mark 8:22–26). Many in the healing ministry today advocate what they call 'soaking prayer'. Ever since the initial ministry from John Wimber and others I have welcomed every opportunity of being prayed for, often with hands laid upon me. Almost every night Anne lays her hands on my liver, curses the cancer in the name of Jesus, and prays for healing. The team has likewise prayed for me frequently, often in very moving ways. I have no doubt about the cumulative effect of this 'soaking prayer'.

Jesus also imparted this healing ministry to others. It was not only to the apostles, although we need to remember that at that time even they were totally inexperienced and often full of unbelief. Jesus also sent out seventy disciples, telling them to heal the sick and to proclaim the Kingdom of God. And those seventy came back thrilled with what they had witnessed: 'Lord, even the demons are subject to us in your name!' (Luke 10:1–20). Moreover it seems from the Great Commission that Christ wanted this ministry to extend to all his disciples: they were to do *all* that he had commanded them, and from his own example this surely would have included healing. Certainly this is how the New Testament Church understood it, and 'many wonders and signs' took place.

In this century there is little doubt that there has been a huge resurgence of spiritual gifts, including healing, in spite of the lack of them for many generations. For too long we have over-intellectualised the Christian faith, reducing much of it to the level of words and propositions. 'Knowing God' has become little more than statements about God – and even here the Church has been cautious and confused.

Others in the Church have been less confused. They fully accept the element of the miraculous in the New Testament, but believe that such expectations for today are foolish in view of the scientific progress that has developed over the years. They rightly reject an unthinking Christianity, and are weary of a simplistic view of healing, which can cause at best disappointed hopes and at worst a total abandonment of faith. Many are struggling honestly with the valid application of biblical teaching to the culture of today, desiring to maintain an intellectual integrity throughout.

So much is valid, providing that once again we do not reduce God to the level of our own understanding. God's thoughts are not our thoughts, and his ways are not our ways. He is infinitely greater than all that we can conceive by human logic or scientific research. We need the Spirit of God to lift our faith until we believe in God who through Jesus forgave sin, cared for the oppressed, healed the sick and cast out demons. *That* is the God in whom we are to believe, and only as we trust him for his power to work today, even when our minds cannot comprehend it, will we see God's kingdom come.

If we really want to see the Kingdom of God amongst us, we must let it begin in our own hearts. We need to bow our wills to Christ's authority and bend our minds to his word. He calls us to love God with all our heart, mind, soul and strength, and to love our neighbours as ourselves. The rule of the kingdom is love, and love learns to trust whether it understands or not. Children do this all the time. They have no difficulty in trusting when their minds are not yet able to comprehend. Although we should become mature in our thinking as Christians, we need a child-like simplicity in our faith in God. It is through this faith, said Jesus, that we enter and enjoy the Kingdom.

16

Is Suffering Punishment?

'How could this happen to you?' Many people have asked me this question. The implication is that there seems to be something unfair about the fact of my cancer. Not only am I a Christian and a clergyman, but I have spent most of my life trying to help people find the love of God – and look at the way I have been rewarded for all my work! To be honest I have never thought in terms of unfairness at all, but others on my behalf have been puzzled, some depressed, and a few even angry.

This raises the greatest and most common objection to belief in God: *the problem of suffering.* I am well aware that in countless other cases the apparent injustices are far more horrific than in my own. Why are tens of thousands of babies born deformed every year? How could God allow millions of innocent and helpless people to die of starvation? For what divine purpose are young parents struck down by fatal diseases, children killed in road accidents, good people swept away by flood or destroyed by fire? How can senseless tragedies cut young people down in their prime of life?

It is worth noting that suffering becomes a problem only when we accept the existence of a good God. The common exclamation 'Good God' is often used when faced suddenly with bad news that is hard to understand. If there is no God, or if God is not good, there is no problem. The universe is nothing more than random choices and meaningless events. There is no fairness, no vindication of right over wrong, no ultimate purposes, no absolute values. 'Man now realises that he is an accident,' said the modern painter Francis Bacon. 'He is a completely futile being (and) has to play out the game without reason.' If there is no 'good God', that is the logical consequence, and to protest about suffering is as foolish as to protest about a number thrown by a dice.

> Life has no reason,
> A struggling through the gloom;
> And the senseless end of it
> Is the insult of the tomb.

If we accept, however, the Judaeo-Christian belief that God is a just God who is all-powerful, all-wise and all-good, we are immediately faced with enormous questions about the vast catalogue of human suffering. Why does God allow it? How could there be any conceivable purpose to it? Even if we could find theoretical answers, these seem to vanish quickly when faced with personal pain, tears and anguish. 'Man is absurd,' wrote Jean-Paul Sartre, 'but he must grimly act as if he were not.' Life becomes little more than gritting one's teeth in the midst of purposeless pain.

Often in the Bible the question of suffering is raised, but nowhere is it so thoroughly developed as in the Book of Job, which Tennyson called 'the greatest poem of ancient or modern times'. We are told at the start of this story that Job is a good and upright man, yet in spite of that he is overwhelmed with appalling tragedies. At first all his animals and servants are either stolen or destroyed. Then his seven sons and three daughters are killed by a devastating tornado. Finally Job himself is smitten with 'loathsome sores from the sole of his foot to the crown of his head'. His appearance becomes so gruesome that his friends scarcely recognise him, and in every way he is tormented with grief and pain.

Understandably Job goes through a wide range of human responses. He loathes himself, is angry with God and finally lapses into self-pity: 'Have pity on me, have pity on me, O you my friends, for the hand of God has touched me!' (19:21).

The burning question posed by the whole book is Why? Why has it happened, if God is still God? Why should a righteous man suffer? Why is there such injustice in the world? *Why?* The rest of the story of Job looks at possible answers to this baffling question. We shall look at some of the less satisfactory explanations in this chapter and the next, and then see if there is anything more helpful to say in the following two. Throughout I shall refer back to my own situation as a reminder that we are considering real people with serious problems, and not merely a philosophical inquiry. These are some of the questions that I have considered carefully, especially over the last few months.

The story unfolds with Job's three comforters who point the finger, not at Job's misfortunes, but at Job himself. Their understanding of the situation is simple but severe: suffering is always due to personal sin. For Job to suffer so acutely, he must surely be guilty of serious sin. Eliphaz the Temanite asks, 'Think now, who that was innocent ever perished? Or where were the upright cut off?' Bildad the Shuhite goes even further by declaring that the calamity falling on Job's family is clear proof of their transgressions, since all godless people will perish. Zophar the Naamathite then puts the final nail in Job's coffin by saying, 'Know then that God exacts of you less than your guilt deserves' (11:6). We see here the origin of the expression 'Job's comforter' which has come to describe someone who only aggravates the distress of the person he is supposed to comfort.

The direct equation of suffering and sin is clearly inadequate and in most cases disastrous. It is seldom as simple as that. In a few cases it may be true of course. Sexual promiscuity may result in venereal disease; over-work may lead to heart attacks; lack of forgiveness, it is thought, may cause or intensify arthritis. Sometimes we have only ourselves to blame for the painful consequences of our sinful actions. Although in the Gospels the implication is rare, on one or two occasions Jesus suggests that sin could have been the basic problem behind a sick person's condition. When a paralysed man was brought before him, the first words that Jesus said to him were, 'My son, your sins are forgiven' (Mark 2:5). Since this man's forgiveness was linked with his healing it is at least possible that his sin was connected with his disease. At another time Jesus healed a man who had been sick for thirty-eight years, and then he said, 'See, you are well! Sin no more, *that nothing worse befall you*' (John 5:14). Here was a serious warning of the solemn consequences of deliberate sin.

In this liberal age we tend naturally to avoid any thought of God's judgment. Yet if we look carefully at the Gospel records we see strong warnings given frequently by Jesus. It is significant that the one person who has shown us more than anyone of the love of God has also told us more than anyone (in the Bible) of the judgment of God. Love risks being rejected. Love will never force. If we don't want God, we won't have God; if we want to be on our own, on our own we shall be, with all its tragic outcome. In Romans 1, Paul talks about those who suppress the truth of God that can be known and who turn their backs on him. Three times Paul writes, 'God gave them up.' If they are determined to live a sinful life, with all its disastrous consequences, God with infinite sadness lets them get on with it. He lets them go or gives them up. It is therefore possible to experience something of God's holy displeasure here and now, if only as a loving warning of the final awesome judgment to come. 'It is a fearful thing to fall into the hands of the living God' (Hebrews 10:31).

Having said all this, in the vast majority of cases it would be quite wrong to link personal suffering with personal sin. When meeting a man born blind, the disciples asked Jesus if this man or his parents had sinned. Jesus replied that neither had been responsible for his blindness: 'He is blind so that God's power might be seen at work in him' (John 9:3, *Good News Bible*). The man was promptly healed.

The danger about coupling suffering with sin is that the sick person may often feel guilty anyway. Many times I have talked with those who are seriously ill, and I have found them anxiously wondering what they had done to bring about their condition. They blame themselves; or if they cannot live with that, they project their guilt on to others or God. It's someone's fault! The trouble is that either feelings of guilt, which are often imaginary, or direct accusations, which are often unfair, only encourage the sickness. Both hinder healing.

Yet I know how easy this is. Sometimes I have thought of my asthma or cancer as being punishment for sin. I remember with shame many foolish things I have done in the past, and with a fairly sensitive conscience it is not hard to feel both guilty and condemned. The positive side is that every affliction has caused me to search deeply within my heart and to repent of every sinful action or attitude that I could discover. I have known many people who have been dramatically healed following such repentance together with the experience of God's forgiveness. It is no bad thing, therefore, to consider carefully our life in the sight of God in order to know the joy and freedom of his love.

At the same time, the negative side of all this comes when such heart-searching leads to nagging and unhealthy feelings of guilt, and perhaps to a very poor image of God. Is it conceivable, when we see Jesus healing the sick and forgiving the sinful, that God should say, 'Ah, there's David Watson. He slipped up rather badly last month so I'll afflict him with asthma for the next twenty years.' Or later, 'He's upset me again, so this time I'll destroy him with cancer.' Such thoughts are not only ridiculous; they are almost blasphemous, and utterly alien to a God of infinite love and mercy as we see him so clearly in Jesus. However, ever since I have had cancer I have often needed the confirmation of God's personal love towards me. In this, the attitude and actions of others have been more important than their words. I am thoroughly aware of my failings and only too willing to believe that my sickness is what I deserve – indeed much less than I deserve. As far as straight justice is concerned that is true. But when I reflect on God's love and mercy in the scriptures I am comforted, especially when that love is *shown* by other Christians around me.

Once when I was deeply depressed, possibly due to a sense of personal failure, a friend wrote to share what he thought God was saying to me, although he knew nothing about my depression at the time.

> My child, I want you to know and feel that I know and love you. I love you because I first knew you. I know you at depths that are even hidden from you. My Spirit searches every corner of your being. I love you, not because I don't know and understand you, but because I do know and understand you. I want you to know and feel that I love you as you are, not because of what you have already achieved for me in my power, not because of what you hope to achieve, but because of who you are, my child. Enjoy who you are, my child; my child who has nothing to prove but the depths of your Father's everlasting and unchanging love.

I took that as a prophetic word, a word from God, and it completely unlocked my depression. I had been blaming myself about some quite trivial matter (I was exhausted at the time), and although I was constantly telling others how much God loved them, I needed to hear and know that for myself.

We assume there must be some cause and effect in suffering, and the sensitive person will quickly suppose that he is to blame for any sickness or tragedy that may come. More than ever, then, others need to reassure that person repeatedly that God loves him just as he is. In the last few months I have received some highly insensitive letters from people I have never met, urging me to repent if I want to be healed. Different sins are specified. Apparently I need to repent for my double-mindedness, for my pride, for my unbelief, and even for being a member of the Anglican Church! No Christian is perfect, of course, and no doubt there is much in my life that still needs purifying. But at a time when my conscience is *over*-sensitive through my illness, more than anything I need to be reminded of God's love. 'Job's comforters', for me, have proved little more than the accusations of Satan. What Job needed (and so did I) was not theology but sympathy, not condemnation but affirmation, not cold moralising but warm compassion. Painful wounds call for love, understanding and healing.

Is Suffering a Test?

'What have I done to deserve this?' No question is more persistent in time of sickness or pain.

Job's comforters eventually retire from the scene (after thirty-one chapters linking suffering with sin!), their accusations having been vigorously refuted by Job. Then comes a much younger man, Elihu, who is diffident about speaking, but is angry with the condemnation of the other three and disappointed with the self-righteousness of Job. He offers a second explanation to suffering.

God is not a judge and executioner, but a teacher. There is a disciplinary and chastening process behind Job's affliction.

> . . . He opens the ears of men,
>   and terrifies them with warnings,
> that he may turn man aside from his deed,
>   and cut off pride from man . . .
> Man is also chastened with pain upon his bed . . .
> Then man prays to God, and he accepts him . . .
>   (33:16–19, 26)

Repeatedly Elihu expounds the same theme:

> If they are bound in fetters
>   and caught in the cords of affliction,
> then he declares to them their work
>   and their transgressions, that they are
>   behaving arrogantly.

He opens their ears to instruction,
  and commands that they return from iniquity.
If they hearken and serve him,
  they complete their days in prosperity,
  and their years in pleasantness.
But if they do not hearken, they perish by the sword,
  and die without knowledge.

(36:8–12)

Constantly God is trying to train and fashion us into his will, and the process may be painful at times. We must humbly accept that he knows what he is doing, and later we will see the value of it.

There is much in the rest of scripture, including the New Testament, to show that Elihu was certainly nearer the mark than the other comforters. In the parable of the vineyard, Jesus said that the gardener *prunes* the fruit-bearing branch 'that it may bear more fruit' (John 15:2). All pruning hurts. 'The Lord disciplines him whom he loves, and chastises every son whom he receives' (Hebrews 12:6). Our faith, said the apostle Peter, may be tested by fire so that one day it may redound to the glory of God (1 Peter 1:7). Paul also referred to a godly grief producing repentance that leads to salvation, and he showed the Corinthian Christians how their suffering led to renewed earnestness and zeal, love and justice (2 Corinthians 7).

There is no doubt that millions of Christians all down the centuries have become more Christ-like through suffering. I know of many who have an almost ethereal beauty about them, refined through pain. In fact those who have experienced more of the love of God than anyone I have ever met have also endured more suffering. When you crush lavender, you find its full fragrance; when you squeeze an orange, you extract its sweet juice. In the same way it is often through pains and hurts that we develop the fragrance and sweetness of Jesus in our lives. An agnostic Professor of Philosophy at Princeton University became a Christian when he studied carefully the lives of some of the great saints of God throughout the history of the Church. What struck him especially was their radiance in the midst of pain. Often they suffered intensely, far more than most other people, yet through all their agony their spirits shone with a glorious lustre that defied extinction. This philosopher became convinced that some power was at work within them, and this discovery eventually brought him to Christ.

In the words of Rabbi Joseph B. Soloveitchik, 'Suffering comes to ennoble man, to purge his thoughts of pride and superficiality, to expand his horizons. In sum, the purpose of suffering is to repair that which is faulty in a man's personality.'[1] Much of that is true, and the examples of courage, faith, patience and compassion that have grown out of suffering are legion. A man who spent over twenty years in Communist prisons in Czechoslovakia where they broke his bones but not his spirit, later referred to those years as the richest of his life. His character was marked by serenity and joy. It is sometimes said that the most distant object we can see in the bright light of day is the sun; but in the dark of night we can see stars which are millions of times further away. Christians down the ages have discovered the 'treasures of darkness' and have gained a richness of maturity and spirituality that would have been impossible when the sun was shining.

It is worth noting, however, that the suffering mentioned in the New Testament that can produce great qualities of spirituality is nearly always that of adversity and persecution. Although the precise interpretation of some passages is debatable, such as Paul's thorn in the flesh, there is little or no reference to sickness as being part of God's chastening process. Too easily we apply the expression of 'taking up our cross' to sickness when originally Jesus meant something

---

[1] Quoted in *When Bad Things Happen to Good People*, Harold S. Kushner, Pan, page 28. (An intriguing book, born out of personal suffering and much counselling, but to my mind extremely unsatisfactory and at times far from the teaching of scripture.)

entirely different. Disease cannot be taken as 'sharing Christ's sufferings'. However, those of us who often visit the sick have surely come away on many occasions with our own faith stimulated by the reality of Christ's love and peace in those who suffer.

Young though he was, Elihu was wise in his comments to Job, but suffering cannot always be explained in its educational and disciplinary effect. What can we say to the mother of a child who has just been killed on the roads? If it was a lesson to be more careful on the roads, the instruction came too late for the child, and it was hardly comforting for the mother. It might have crippled her with guilt. The lesson was altogether too expensive. Rabbi Harold S. Kushner makes a fair point when he says, 'I am offended by those who suggest that God creates retarded children so that those around them will learn compassion and gratitude. Why should God distort someone else's life to such a degree in order to enhance my spiritual sensitivity?' Elihu's theory of discipline is right in some cases, but it becomes bizarre in others. Could the God who revealed himself so perfectly in Jesus conceivably invent such a callous system of moral education? And if the Lord genuinely loves those whom he chastens, could he inflict such appalling suffering on innocent children for the purpose of loving correction?

A refinement of Elihu's teaching is that God allows suffering for a test. The classic illustration of this is in the story of Abraham and Isaac (Genesis 22). Abraham was told by God to sacrifice his only son Isaac, and he obeyed right up to the point of raising his knife to plunge it into the body of his son. Isaac's life was spared by God at the last moment, but this was the ultimate test of Abraham's faith, and therefore God was able to trust him with much blessing. It is significant that those whom God has unusually blessed down the ages have also endured unusual pain, often some form of persecution but other afflictions as well. The twentieth century prophet, A. W. Tozer, once wrote: 'It is doubtful if God can bless a man greatly without hurting him deeply.' The apostle Peter

also told his readers not to be surprised by the 'fiery ordeal'
which would soon come upon them. He told them to rejoice
in sharing Christ's sufferings 'because the Spirit of glory and
of God rests upon you' (1 Peter 4:12–14). Blessings and
buffetings usually go hand in hand.

The whole story of Job, too, could be seen as a test. In the
prologue (chapters 1 and 2), Satan comes before God and is
given permission to afflict Job in any way he wants, up to a
certain point. After the first catastrophe concerning his
possessions and family, Job is still able to declare, 'The Lord
gave, and the Lord has taken away; blessed be the name of
the Lord.' Satan comes back again, and this time God gives
him permission to smite Job's body, but not to take away his
life. Job initially stands up to the test once again, and says
submissively, 'Shall we receive good at the hand of God, and
shall we not receive evil?' Later, however, the wretched
discomfort of his disease undermines his peace and he begins
to curse the day of his birth. The rest of the book effectively
asks the question, 'If suffering is allowed by God as a test of
our faith, why does he do it? What is to be gained by it? Is it
really necessary?'

One or two people have said to me that God must love and
trust me very much to test me with an inoperable cancer. I
have never replied to them, partly because I question the
theology on which they base their remarks and partly because, if they were right, I frankly wish that God did not trust
me so much! I would be quite content with less trust on his
part and less suffering on mine. It would be a curious way of
showing his love to me, and I cannot imagine that I could
even think of inflicting such a thing on my children, had I the
power to do so.

A more serious objection to this viewpoint is that numerous people suffer far more acutely than I have ever done, and
many of them have clearly been crushed by the test. As a
result of their pain they have suffered nervous breakdowns,
their marriages have broken up or they have become bitter
atheists. If suffering is to be regarded purely as a test of our

faith, God at times seems to have miscalculated wildly.

The attempted answers to suffering that we have seen so far are therefore inadequate, even if they hold important elements of truth. In the next chapters we shall see if there is anything more to be said and if we are even asking the right questions.

18

What is God saying to me?

During the last few months I have felt extremely vulnerable.
Unexplained aches and pains all too easily appear sinister.
For the last three months, for example, I have had increasing
backache – a common complaint but something I have never
known in my life. Has the cancer gone round to my spine?
What exactly is going on? Both my doctor and specialist say
that in their opinion it is purely muscular and postural. But
the pain continues, especially when I am standing (as I often
am), and I wonder why? Why *now*? It is an easy temptation to
fear the worst.

Then the tumour in my liver, which for the first time I
could feel a few weeks ago, began to harden and became
sore – so sore, in fact, that I could sleep only in one position.
Again, what was going on? In one difficult week recently, my
specialist thought that the tumour in the liver was definitely
growing, but three days later my surgeon was sure that it was
not growing – if anything slightly smaller and softer.

During this period we had special times of prayer for my
healing. They were always extremely helpful. The sore, hard
lump is no longer sore (and much softer), but the pains in my
back seem to get worse – for whatever reason.

Walking by faith is rather like walking on a tight-rope: at
times it is exhilarating, but it requires only the slightest
knock to make me feel insecure and anxious. In the last week
or so I have been bothered more by asthma, which probably
indicates an increased level of stress. I have also not been
sleeping so well as before.

I mention all this, not to wallow in self-pity (I *still* believe that God is healing me) but to emphasise that the question 'why suffering?' is far from theoretical. I am profoundly aware that many millions in the world are suffering much more acutely than I am, yet the pains and vulnerability are still there.

For those who believe in a good God, the dilemma is so acute, that Rabbi Kushner concludes that God cannot be all powerful after all. Using the analogy of quantum physics where it seems that certain events happen in the universe at random, Kushner believes that there is 'randomness in the universe . . . Why do we have to insist on everything being reasonable? Why can't we let the universe have a few rough edges?'[1] According to Kushner, God is not in control of everything, although he is on our side whenever bad luck dominates. Evil sometimes finally prevails and is not always overcome by good. Kushner claims that God does not have the whole world in his hands, and therefore is not responsible for malformed children, for natural disasters, or fatal diseases. These simply lie outside his jurisdiction.

It is a neat theory, and it saves us from the unacceptable conclusion of blaming God for all the evil in the world. However, if God is not in ultimate control, he cannot truly be God. If there is no final justice, no eventual triumph of good over evil, God is not the God who has revealed himself in the Bible and in the person of Jesus Christ. If there is some whimsical evil force greater than God, making God finite and limited, we live a futile existence in a meaningless world – as the atheist maintains. If God is not God of all, he is not God at all. There is little hope for any of us, apart from resigning ourselves to a fortuitous mortality in a universe ruled by chance. We cannot ultimately be sure of anything except being at the mercy of unleashed and unpredictable evil.

However, the ringing conviction of the scriptures is that *the*

[1] *When Bad Things Happen to Good People*

Lord reigns! Even in the one supreme case of truly innocent suffering, the crucifixion of Jesus, God knew what he was doing. He had not lost control. As Simon Peter declared, all the rulers put together could do only what God had planned to take place (Acts 4:27f:). At the time no one could see why such excruciating suffering should destroy the only sinless man that had ever lived, the Son of God himself. Later the disciples saw it as clearly as could be. 'Christ died for our sins once for all,' wrote Peter. 'He the just suffered for the unjust, to bring us to God' (1 Peter 3:18, *New English Bible*). There on the cross Christ bore the penalty for our sin once for all, so that we might be reconciled to God.

Nevertheless, although Christians down the ages have seen in Christ's sufferings the salvation of the world, what can we say about the myriads of others whose sufferings and death have never had any special significance, or none that we could discern?

James Mitchell in *The god I want* once wrote angrily: 'The value of a god must be open to test. No god is worth preserving unless he is of some practical use in curing all the ills which plague humanity – all the disease and pain and starvation, the little children born crippled or spastic or mentally defective: a creator god would be answerable to *us* for these things at the day of judgment – if he dared to turn up.' Here is the bitter anger that many feel towards God when faced with senseless and hopeless suffering.

Interestingly enough we find many expressions of anger against God in the Psalms. The psalmist often reveals the deepest hurts of his heart, whether they are godly or not.

> Why dost thou stand far off, O Lord?
> Why dost thou hide thyself in times of trouble?
>
> (Psalm 10:1)

> My God, my God, why hast thou forsaken me?
> Why art thou so far from helping me, from the words of
>   my groaning?

O my God, I cry by day, but thou dost not answer;
and by night, but find no rest.

(Psalm 22:1f)

My tears have been my food day and night,
While men say to me continually, 'Where is your God?'

(Psalm 42:3)

Here are some cries taken almost at random from the Psalms. Similar quotations are numerous. It is worth mentioning that when we feel angry, bitter, helpless or in despair, it is good to be honest with God about our feelings. In fact, it is much better expressing our anguish *to* God than talking resentfully *about* God to others. God can take on anger. Indeed he did take our anger and all our other sins when his Son died on the cross for us. He wants us to be honest with him and not to put on a pious mask when we approach him.

At the same time, the psalmist in Psalm 73, having complained bitterly about his continuous suffering, comes humbly to realise that his attitude to God was all wrong:

When my thoughts were bitter
and my feelings were hurt,
I was as stupid as an animal;
I did not understand you . . .
What else have I in heaven but you?
Since I have you, what else could I
want on earth?
My mind and my body may grow weak,
but God is my strength;
he is all I ever need . . .

(vv 21–26, *Good News Bible*)

Behind much anger about suffering is our human arrogance which assumes that God must somehow justify his existence and explain his actions before we are prepared to consider the possibility of believing in him.

Sometimes I am asked, 'Is God relevant to me?' But that is

not the crucial question at all. A much more vital issue is this: 'Am I relevant to God?' The astonishing answer is that each of us is incredibly relevant to an infinite God of love who is with us in all our afflictions and wants to deliver us from negative reactions to those afflictions. In our natural self-centredness we tend to think that we are at the centre of the universe, and that God (if he exists at all) is there simply to meet our needs. We regard him as a servant whom we call in from time to time to clear up the mess we are in – a mess often of our own doing. But we are not at the centre of the universe. God is. And God is not our servant. He is our Lord. The question is not 'Why should I bother with God?' but 'Why should God bother with me?' That is a much harder question to answer. There is no reason why God should bother with me at all, since I have so often turned my back on him. But he does. For God is love. Sometimes it is only through suffering that our self-importance is broken. We need humbly to realise our own smallness and sinfulness in contrast to God's greatness and holiness.

Franklin D. Roosevelt, when President of the United States of America, used to have a little ritual with the naturalist William Beebe. After dinner together, the two men would go outside and look up into the night-sky. They would find the lower left-hand corner of the great square of Pegasus. One of them would then recite these words: 'That is the spiral galaxy of Andromeda. It is as large as our Milky Way. It is one of a hundred million galaxies. It is 750,000 light years away. It consists of a hundred billion suns, each one larger than our sun.' They would then pause for a few moments, and Roosevelt would finally say, 'Now I think we feel small enough! Let's go to bed!' Although man has great dignity, being made in the image of God, he must also appreciate his smallness and his natural inability to grasp more than a tiny fraction of total reality.

This was the substance of God's answer to Job. In four great chapters God gently challenged Job as to how much he understood about God and his ways of working. Humbly at the end of it all, Job realised that he knew virtually nothing, and his demand to fathom all the answers to his suffering was both foolish and unreasonable. 'I have uttered what I did not understand,' he said. 'I despise myself, and repent in dust and ashes.' Then God began to bless him once again.

Some will not find this satisfactory. Together with our suffering, they will say, do we also have to be browbeaten by God into submission? Is that the moral of the story? We should not think of it like that. If we have any conception of the greatness of God we should refrain from pressing the question *Why?* however understandable that might be. On many thousands of issues we simply do not and cannot know. Why does God allow the birth of severely handicapped children? I don't know. Why are some individuals plagued with tragedies for much of their lives, whilst others suffer hardly at all? I don't know. Why is there seeming injustice on every side? I don't know. The questions are endless if we ask why? Instead we should ask the question *What?* 'What are you saying to me, God? What are you doing in my life? What response do you want me to make?' With that question we can expect an answer.

It is my conviction that God is always trying to speak to us in his love, even when his word is hard to accept. 'Man shall not live by bread alone,' said Jesus, 'but by every word that proceeds from the mouth of God.' This was a quotation from the Old Testament which Jesus used when being tempted by his adversary in the wilderness. More important than anything is knowing God's will and doing it. It is far more important than having intellectual answers to all our philosophical questions about God and man, suffering and pain. Life anyway is short and uncertain, but God's word endures for ever. However, our lives are often so full of other things that we find it impossible to hear or discern what God is saying to us. Our ears are deaf, our minds dull and our wills stubborn. We do not hear God speak, or if we do, we fail to respond.

It is sometimes only through suffering that we begin to listen to God. Our natural pride and self-confidence have been stripped painfully away, and we become aware, perhaps for the first time, of our own personal needs. We may even begin to ask God for help instead of protesting about our condition or insisting on explanations. I have met several people who do not profess any commitment to Christ who still pray when facing suffering.

During the ministry of Jesus on earth, a tower fell in Siloam and killed eighteen innocent people. 'Why did God allow it?' was the immediate question pressed by those around him. We may have exactly the same question when we hear of accidents, earthquakes and disasters every day in the news. Jesus replied, not by answering the vexed question of suffering nor by giving a satisfactory solution to this particular tragedy. As perfect Man, accepting our human limitations, Jesus may not even have known the reason why. Instead he came back to the practical challenge of God's word: 'I tell you . . . unless you repent you will all likewise perish' (Luke 13:1–5). It may sound a little bleak, but Jesus was far more concerned with a person's eternal well-being than merely satisfying an intellectual curiosity. Here he was dealing not with the question of Why? but with the question What? What is God saying in this calamity? It is a reminder that life in this world is frail and uncertain. We cannot boast of tomorrow. It is therefore vital that we sort out our relationship with God here and now. Then we are ready for anything. 'Teach us to number our days,' prayed the psalmist 'that we may get a heart of wisdom' (Psalm 90:12).

Through the unexpected diagnosis of cancer I was forced to consider carefully my priorities in life and to make some necessary adjustments. I still do not know why God allowed it, nor does it bother me. But I am beginning to hear what God is saying, and this has been enormously helpful to me. As I turn to the Bible, I find passages coming alive for me, perhaps more than ever before. As I praise God or listen to worship cassettes, my vision of the greatness and love of God is being continually reinforced. I am content to trust myself to a loving God whose control is ultimate and whose wisdom transcends my own feeble understanding.

C. S. Lewis once put it graphically like this: 'God is the only comfort, he is also the supreme terror: the thing we most need and the thing we most want to hide from. He is our only ally, and we have made ourselves his enemies. Some people talk as if meeting the gaze of Absolute Goodness would be fun. They need to think again!' God is so concerned that we should know his love that he will sometimes speak to us in severe terms if we will not listen to him in any other way. The suffering may be ours or that of someone else whom we know and love. Whatever it is, we should think carefully about what God is trying to say to us. C. S. Lewis elsewhere emphasises that it is a poor thing if we turn to God *only* in suffering, *only* because there is nothing better to be had. 'It is hardly complimentary to God that we should choose him as an alternative to hell; yet even this he accepts. The creature's illusions of self-sufficiency must, for the creature's sake, be shattered.'[2] Humbly we need to learn that because God is love, there is the awful possibility of neglecting and forfeiting his love, and at the same time he offers us the unspeakable joy of knowing that love in our own experience, perhaps especially in the midst of suffering.

Joni (pronounced Johnny) Eareckson, as an athletic young girl of seventeen broke her neck when diving into the sea and has been totally paralysed from the neck down ever since. She suffered considerably during her lengthy periods in hospital, and even as a deeply committed Christian found herself asking, often with anger and frustration, the question Why? A wise friend said this to her: 'You don't have to know why God let you be hurt. The fact is, God knows – and that's all that counts. Just trust him to work things out for good, eventually, if not right away.'

'What do you mean?' asked Joni.

[2] *The Problem of Pain*, Bles.

'Would you be any happier if you did know why God wants you paralysed? I doubt it. So don't get worked up trying to find meaning to the accident.'[3]

If we insist on pursuing the question Why? we shall only increase our sense of frustration and perhaps bitterness. We only add to our injury and block the way for God's love to reach us.

Michel Quoist has expressed it well in one of his *Prayers of Life*.[4] He imagined God speaking to him:

> Son I am here.
> I haven't left you,
> How weak is your faith!
> You are too proud.
> You still rely on yourself . . .
> You must surrender yourself to me.
> You must realise that you are neither
>   big enough or strong enough.
> You must let yourself be guided like a child.
> My little child.
> Come, give me your hand, and do not fear.
> If there is mud, I will carry you in my arms.
> But you must be very very little,
> For the Father carries only little children.

It is this quiet, restful, child-like trust in the Father of love that will enable us to experience his peace, even in the very worst of storms.

[3] *Joni* by Joni Eareckson, Pickering and Inglis, 1976.
[4] Published by Gill and Macmillan Limited, 1963.

19

Overcoming Suffering

Two fathers came to see me within a space of a few months. Each had lost a young child tragically. One child, aged four, had died of leukaemia; the other, aged five, had been drowned in a swimming pool in their own back garden. One father had been a professing Christian before the disaster but became a bitter and militant atheist as a result; the other had been a professing humanist but became a committed Christian as a result. They both had roughly the same suffering to contend with, but their reactions were widely different. One had his bitterness to endure as well as his suffering, which in the long run might well have been worse – it was certainly worse for other people; the other found the peace and love of Christ, which transformed his suffering. In all our afflictions, it is not so much our situation that counts but the way in which we react to it. And our reactions can affect, to a remarkable degree, the outcome of our lives.

I remember meeting a woman who had been a severe and chronic schizophrenic living permanently in a mental hospital. As a young girl she had been sexually assaulted, and each counselling session returned to this nightmare in her past. A Christian minister visited her and surprisingly challenged her about her attitudes, 'You are full of self-pity; self-pity is a form of pride. Unless you repent of your pride you will never be healed.' The woman was understandably furious. However, although she was clearly not responsible for her tragic suffering as a young girl, she *was* responsible for her present responses to that suffering. Slowly she began to repent.

Within a year she was healed and out of hospital. Later she went as a Christian missionary to the Arctic.

Pat Seed, a woman in her fifties, was told a few years ago that she had cancer and only six months to live. Instead of resigning herself to her situation (which would almost certainly have resulted in an early death), she immediately embarked on a fund-raising campaign in order to buy a sophisticated scanner for the early detection of cancer, for the Christie Hospital in Manchester. She worked so hard at this that she scarcely had time to think about anything else, including her own terminal illness. She not only outlived her six months; today, six years later, she has raised more than three million pounds for life-saving equipment. She has been presented with an MBE by the Queen at Buckingham Palace, and she has now been declared entirely free from cancer. Moreover, over 5,000 patients have now been scanned by the equipment bought through her fund-raising, and probably many lives saved. Because she reacted positively to her situation she was able to change it radically. Pat Seed made this interesting comment in a newspaper interview: 'I heard about two cancer patients, both men, who like me were given six months to live. One went home, made arrangements for his funeral, and died a fortnight later. The other went home, looked at his seven children and thought: "How on earth will this lot cope if I go?" Now twenty years later, those children have grown up and he's still alive.'[1] Repeatedly it comes back to our attitudes, which are often more important than the affliction itself.

I too have felt it right to plunge myself into my work, although making a few adjustments where necessary. Although I tire more easily than before, I have been preaching, writing, broadcasting and travelling to a considerable extent. At times my programme has been too full and I have occasionally been trapped by the demands and expectations of others. More firmly than ever I am learning

---

[1] Quoted in the *Daily Mail*, May 26th, 1983.

to say 'No'. However, I am far from inactive and my diary is full for the best part of a year ahead. I certainly have as much work as most people could manage.

'David, you're crazy! You're doing too much!' say some of my friends.

'I agree. I have been pushing it too hard recently. But often I spend a quiet evening with my family and I firmly keep one day off a week!' Then I look through my diary to see if I could cancel one or two engagements. Both Hilary and Anne have been invaluable in trying to protect me from unnecessary work, however 'fruitful' it might be.

It is not always easy working hard when in the back of my mind I am conscious of the continuing battle against cancer, backache and asthma. Yet I have not the slightest doubt that a positive attitude to the present and active planning for the future can both aid the healing process. I have also been aware of a greater knowledge of God over these months, and people tell me that there is a new authority in my ministry.

Suffering can often produce great depths of character, mature understanding, warm compassion and rich spirituality. Of course we should always strive to heal the sick and relieve the oppressed; and we should rejoice that in heaven we shall finally be set free from all pains and tears. But suffering can make us more like Christ. The sparkling radiance of a diamond is caused by a lump of coal subjected to extreme pressure and heat over a long period of time. Again, a beautiful pearl emerges when an oyster has to cover an irritating object with layer upon layer of smooth mother-of-pearl lining excreted from its own body. When we suffer in various ways, God is able to use all the pressures and irritations to reveal something of his radiance and beauty in our lives.

God never promises to save us from adversity, only to be with us in the midst of it. Richard Wurmbrand is a Rumanian pastor who endured fourteen years in various Communist prisons, where he was repeatedly tortured for his faith in Christ. 'They broke four vertebrae in my back and many other bones. They carved me in a dozen places. They burned me and cut eighteen holes in my body.' For three years he was in solitary confinement thirty feet below ground level, during which time the only persons he saw were his torturers. In despair he asked God to speak to him, to say something to him. At that moment he heard a terrible piercing cry. It was from another unfortunate victim who was being tortured. But Wurmbrand heard it as a cry from God's heart. God was revealing what he felt like when he saw his children in pain. 'In all their affliction he was afflicted' (Isaiah 63:9). God shares in our suffering. In that filthy underground prison Wurmbrand discovered a beauty in Christ that he had not known before. He literally danced for joy.

God can do anything, and theoretically could have programmed us as robots, impervious to pain and unable to inflict it on others. Had he done so, life might have been simpler, but there would also have been no feeling, no freedom, no relationships, no love – nothing of those human qualities which make life worth living. Instead, God has made us with a genuine freedom of choice to go his way or ours; and because we have all naturally gone our way instead of his, we live in a fallen world which is still often staggeringly beautiful but which is sadly marred by sin, suffering and death. God has therefore entered our world in Christ and suffers with us.

William Temple once put it like this: ' "There cannot be a God of love," men say, "because if there was, and he looked upon the world, his heart would break." The Church points to the Cross and says, "It did break," "It is God who made the world," men say. "It is he who should bear the load." The Church points to the Cross and says, "He did bear it." ' Although Christ has suffered once-for-all on the cross for our sins, he still today weeps with those who weep, he feels our pain and enters into our sorrows with his compassionate love.

This raises a very important point. I have been acutely aware of the unusual privileges I have received – perhaps because of my writing and preaching around the world. Not every cancer-sufferer will have pastors flying over from California to see him. Not everyone afflicted will have the benefit of many thousands praying. Why should I be a special case?

The flat answer, of course, is that I am not. God is no respecter of persons, and loves each person equally with his immeasurable, steadfast love. In human terms, that love will naturally vary in expression. But God's unfailing love is the one constancy that everyone of us can trust.

We need also to realise that God's love was most perfectly portrayed *through* the supreme suffering of Jesus on the cross. That intensity of suffering is, almost paradoxically, the measure of God's love. God, in his love, may not spare us from severe suffering (there is no guarantee that he will spare me or anyone else reading this book). But even when everything seems dark, painful, desperate and hopeless, God still loves, is still there, and will never fail us. The cross is the ultimate proof of that.

The prayer for the sick in the Alternative Service Book for the Church of England puts it well:

Heavenly Father,
giver of life and health:
comfort and restore those who are sick,
that they may be strengthened in their weakness
and have confidence in your unfailing love;
through Jesus Christ our Lord.

More often than not we cannot find answers to suffering, if by answers we mean explanations. Why did the plane crash? Why did a loved one die of cancer? Why was that child killed on the roads? We may never find a satisfying explanation, and the danger is that we may end up blaming someone, either ourselves or God. There are seldom good *reasons* for suffering, but there can be good *responses*. I am not suggesting

that such good responses are easy. Far from it. For me it has
often been an act of the will to listen to worship cassettes, to
read the scriptures, to receive communion, to join in with
other Christians, to pray and praise and to meditate on the
sufferings of Christ. However the more I make myself aware
of God's love (whether I *feel* his love or not – usually I don't),
the more God can change my negatives into positives. It is a
battle, especially at night, but it is certainly important.
Unless I eat physically, I waste away; and unless I 'feed
spiritually' in ways I have described, I submerge in the
seductive sea of self-pity.

As we learn to respond positively, however, we shall be
able, one way or another, to overcome suffering so that the
explanation becomes no longer of major importance. Those
who learn that lesson often achieve a remarkable quality of
life that may be far in excess of the trouble-free existence of
others. It is not what we *do*, but who we *are* that matters most
in life; and it is not *what* we endure, but the *way* we endure it
that counts. We can overcome evil with good.

Jesus clearly warned us not to build all our hopes and
happiness on this life. Inevitably we live in a fallen, evil
world, and one day we stand to lose everything except those
qualities that have eternal value. He urged us again and
again to lay up for ourselves treasures in heaven, 'where
neither moth nor rust consumes and where thieves do not
break in and steal' (Matthew 6:20). There is no immunity
promised to anyone from the pains and sorrows of this world,
but we are to be confident in our hope that the best is yet to
be.

The author of Lamentations in the Old Testament once
felt utterly crushed by his sufferings: 'My soul is bereft of
peace, I have forgotten what happiness is,' he said. He was
'bowed down' within himself – until he deliberately, as an
act of the will, called this truth to mind and so stimulated his
hope:

> The steadfast love of the Lord never ceases,
>   his mercies never come to an end;
> they are new every morning;
>   great is thy faithfulness.
> 'The Lord is my portion,' says my soul,
>   'therefore I will hope in him.'
>
>   (3:22–24)

Looking positively towards the future has helped me in my present need. Since my life is in the hands of God, I am able to trust that God's love is always there and God's plan is always good.

Throughout the centuries, a strong hope for the future has kept God's people firm in their faith in the midst of appalling anguish. The apostle Paul wrote, 'I consider that the sufferings of this present time are not worth comparing with the glory that is to be revealed to us' (Romans 8:18). Elsewhere he talked about being 'afflicted . . . perplexed . . . persecuted . . . struck down', and yet he could write, 'For this slight momentary affliction is preparing for us an eternal weight of glory beyond all comparison' (2 Corinthians 4:17). If we look at the eleventh chapter of that letter we see what 'slight momentary affliction' Paul was referring to:

> Five times I have received at the hands of the Jews the forty lashes less one. Three times I have been beaten with rods; once I was stoned. Three times I have been shipwrecked; a night and a day I have been adrift at sea; on frequent journeys, in danger from rivers, danger from robbers, danger from my own people, danger from Gentiles, danger in the city, danger in the wilderness, danger at sea, danger from false brethren; in toil and hardship, through many a sleepless night, in hunger and thirst, often without food, in cold and exposure . . .
>
>   (2 Corinthians 11:24–27)

Yet compared with the 'eternal weight' of God's glory, all this catalogue of suffering was as nothing. The secret was that Paul kept his eyes on the eternal perspective, and this put all his personal agonies and anxieties into proportion. 'We look not to the things that are seen but to the things that are unseen; for the things that are seen are transient, but the things that are unseen are eternal.' Without this dimension of eternity and without a strong hope in heaven, the problems of our human existence might fill us all with despair. But once we know the love of God for ourselves and believe in life after death – or life *through* death – our outlook on this life, with all its pains and sorrows, can be transformed.

Not everyone, however, shares that confidence. Rabbi Kushner writes, 'Because we so desperately want to believe that God will be fair to us, we fasten our hopes on the idea that life in this world is not the only reality . . . (But) neither I nor any other living person can know anything about the reality of that hope.'[2] If left to our own wisdom, that would be true. But the coming of Christ to this world, his clear teaching about the future, his death for our sins and his resurrection from the dead (with all the massive evidence for that), alters the whole situation. We are not left without hope. We *can* know something about life after death. We have good reasons for our faith, solid historical reasons. We can know the risen Christ here and now. For the Christian, the future will be glorious, and that changes our whole attitude to present suffering. If we think of this world only, we have difficulties. But if we see that neither distress nor death can separate us from the love of God, we have a living hope which transcends all the trials of our present existence.

When I was recently in Montreal I met a wonderful black Christian from Uganda called Henry. Henry was one day travelling with his friends on a bus in Uganda when they were ambushed by guerrillas. Shots were fired and Henry had half his face blown away, from the nose downwards. It

[2] *When Bad Things Happen To Good People.*

was a miracle that he survived at all. A Christian organisation called World Vision paid for him to go to Montreal, a city famous for its outstanding medical school, and covered the fees necessary to rebuild Henry's face. When I first saw him he had many more operations to come, and I could not help flinching when I saw the mask that had once been a face. His eyes, however, still sparkled. Since Henry was quite unable to speak he wrote these words: 'God never promises us an easy time. Just a safe arrival.' That is the hope that has kept Henry in God's peace throughout his terrible experience.

It is the hope that all those in Christ can enjoy.

20

Getting Going Again

As I stood up to preach it was an astonishing sight. It was my first sermon since my illness, and I was more than usually nervous. Holy Trinity Brompton, a lively Anglican church in central London with a large and youthful congregation, was packed out. Normally the church seats about 1,000, but extra chairs were out and many were standing at the back and round the side aisles. For good reasons, no publicity had been given about my preaching, so I did not presume that the crowds were there because of me! At the last minute I agreed to preach on May 15th instead of a member of their staff, and I was given the theme: 'The Health of the Kingdom'.

'I confess that I'm a little nervous standing here,' I began. 'But first of all I want to thank you all, more than I can possibly say, for all your prayers over the past months. I wish I could thank you all personally, but I am profoundly grateful – and, thank God, I am feeling very fit.'

I went on to give the precise situation, medically speaking, and encouraged them to continue praying if they wished to do so. I then spoke on the healing ministry of Jesus and the New Testament Church, when the Kingdom of God was both demonstrated and proclaimed with power. At the end I offered some suggestions as to why we did not see more healings in the western Church today, concluding with an exhortation to trust God's word and Spirit, and to get cracking! I knew that many in that church, like me, had been inspired by the teaching and ministry of John Wimber (as well as others), and were already actively praying for people

after almost every evening service. I went forward myself
that night for further prayer.

I loved being back at work again, and I made it my
determination to go on preaching Christ, unfolding as many
of his 'unsearchable riches' as I had yet discovered, for as
long as God gave me health and strength. I was also deeply
moved when John Collins, the Vicar of that church, once
again called the congregation to prayer and fasting on my
behalf.

In those summer months I began to travel again, although
only in short bursts. I went to a Sales Conference in the Lake
District organised by Hodder and Stoughton for their staff. I
went to a dinner at my College in Cambridge, St John's,
meeting friends whom I had not seen for over twenty-five
years. On the way there, I visited a clergyman who was dying
of cancer and prayed with him. I heard only this week that he
has been getting steadily better ever since, even though no
one expected him to live beyond May (five months ago now).
Repeatedly I found, wherever I went, that my illness gave me
immediate opportunities to talk about Christ, my experience
of his love, my belief in his healing and my hopes for the
future. Now when people ask me 'How are you?' I answer
frankly: 'I'm feeling pretty well, thanks. But in fact I've got
cancer.'

This unexpected reply to a conventional greeting has led to
many excellent conversations about basic issues concerning
life and death, God and faith, and I have been thankful not to
be trapped in the usual irrelevant chit-chat which dominates
so many social functions.

A further milestone was reached when I started working
with the team again. Anne and I had missed enormously our
daily meetings with them, although these had recently begun
again whenever they were in London. However, in July, I
returned with the team to Dartford, where we had led an
excellent Christian festival in the Orchard Theatre the previous September – each night throughout the week the
theatre having been completely full. On this occasion we

were there for two nights, and were told that the theatre
could have been filled three times over. I knew once again
that many of those present had been praying for me throughout the year, so the sense of thanksgiving and praise was
excellent. It was marvellous being back there again and even
more so being with the team. When talking with each
member of the team privately I was amazed – and delighted – to discover that all were willing to commit themselves to
this work for another year, although they knew that a risk of
faith was involved in this.

The next week I recorded seven late-night programmes for
TV South, called *Company*. I liked the format of these, with
three people sitting round a kitchen table having a cup of tea
or coffee, chatting about various topics, with the camera
'eavesdropping' on the conversation. Since I was the guest
for the week, much of the discussion centred round my illness
and reactions to it, and the relevance of Christ in every
situation. Everyone seemed pleased with the resulting programmes.

Within a few days I was off again, this time with both my
family and my team, to lead a Families' Christian House-
party, with about 130 people of all ages coming from different
parts of the country. None of us wanted to go! Fiona and Guy
feared that it might be a week of solid and intense religion,
Anne disliked houseparties that were not part of the life of our
own local church, and I shared the misgivings of the team
that this was not the same style as our usual work.

In fact we all had a marvellous week, even if we were
exhausted at the end of it. These houseparties had been well
established by the organisers for a number of years, so we
were thankfully not responsible for the administration. But
the team excelled with the teenagers; and, as usual, they
illustrated my talks in a delightful way with their worship,
drama, mime and dance. 'Can we go again next year?' was
the first question Guy and Fiona asked when we drove away.

I was also thankful that my health had sustained my first
full and fairly intensive week. I had to teach at least twice a

day, counselling individuals in between. Apart from the beginnings of backache and the danger of getting overtired, I felt remarkably well.

Four days later we were off to York for the start of our family holiday. Emotionally neither Anne nor I could have gone to York any earlier. Having lived and worked there for seventeen years, our roots had gone very deep and the tender transplant into London had been in constant danger of 'rejection' over the past year. Although we were not yet settled in London, we felt that we could at least meet those whom we had known and loved so much without being emotionally overwhelmed by it all.

It was wonderful being there, however. I knew how much they had suffered and prayed because of my illness, and just to be there to say 'thank you' was a marvellous experience for us. We loved the gentle and sensitive worship in the church services – a quality of worship that has melted many hearts in the past because it conveys the gentle, healing love of God. Conversations were inevitably brief, but even a minute or two with those who had been especially close to us, were full of silent eloquence. When you love someone deeply, you don't have to *say* very much. Even trivial comments convey a depth of feeling that is mutually understood.

On the Sunday night I preached. I must have preached many hundreds of sermons in that church, St Michael-le-Belfrey, next to York Minster. But this time it was a special, never-to-be-forgotten occasion. In spite of a cloudburst and torrential rain for over an hour before the service, the church was bulging at the seams with people. The seating capacity of the church is approximately 700, but it was estimated that well over 1,000 were present that evening. It was tremendous looking round to see so many with whom I had shared my life deeply in the past. When people have experienced many joys and pains together over the years, there is a depth of fellowship between them that nothing can destroy.

I preached, and Anne prophesied, giving clear directions for the church which confirmed the growing convictions of

the leaders. And the service ended. Not quite. I stood at the
door for about an hour and a half saying goodbye to each of
the 1,000 or more present, shaking hands, hugging or kissing,
whatever seemed appropriate. I thought of the farewell given
to the apostle Paul by the Ephesian elders: 'They all wept
and embraced Paul and kissed him.' To experience the godly
love of God's family is one of the most treasured riches for
those in Christ. If heaven is like this, only much more so, why
are we so reluctant to go there?

It was not yet heaven, however, since my back was almost
killing me after all that standing!

The next day we drove up to Scotland (my back still very
sore) leaving the morning mists in York, and tasting the
unspoilt beauty of the Western Highlands, from the long
sweep of Loch Lomond through the threatening crags of
Glencoe into the towering majesty of Ben Nevis. Our destina-
tion was Glenfinnan, where Bonnie Prince Charlie once
summoned his supporters before marching south to claim the
throne.

Good friends of ours had lent us their lodge in Glenfinnan,
and we joined forces with the Saunders family for ten days in
one of the most beautiful settings imaginable. My back was
causing persistent trouble, which considerably curtailed my
movements apart from a geriatric stroll once a day. But Anne
was in her element, rising at the crack of dawn (almost) to
exercise her puppy in the fresh Scottish air, with the early
mists lifting up the mountains as the sun began to shine
through. Guy spent successful hours by a small loch, pulling
out one rainbow trout after another, which we all enjoyed for
breakfast. Fiona did nothing very energetic, spending most of
her time reading or playing cards with members of the
Saunders family. It was altogether a very good holiday,
rounded off with a few days visiting the great castles of
Northumberland and another brief visit to York, before
returning to London.

For a couple of days John and Carol Wimber came to see
us again, on their return from Sweden to the States, to find

out what progress I was making. All the outward signs of the cancer were good. My blood tests were normal. I was working hard, eating well and sleeping soundly (most of the time).

'My back however is hurting quite a bit,' I said. 'I would be glad if you would pray for it.'

'Sure, we often pray for backs and we never have any problems!' replied John with a twinkle in his eye.

John, Carol and Anne prayed. We all believed that God had heard our prayer. But nothing happened! My back continued to be just as painful as before. Why? I don't know. I do know that countless backs and many more serious problems have been healed by Christ through the ministry of John and others. Sometimes the cause of the pain is healed instantly. Sometimes it is a much more drawn-out battle. Once again, we may not understand the reasons for this, but we can make the right responses. I continued to thank God that he was at work, healing my back and releasing me from cancer.

This time John asked another pastor to see us, Kenn Gullickson and his wife Joni. We had met Kenn and Joni before, and knew that God had given them a special ministry of healing life's hurts. All of us have inner and often deep-seated hurts due to our past experiences. What we may not always consciously realise is that these wounds can leave behind equally deep-seated areas of resentment or bitterness. On the surface we may not be aware of anything wrong, but hidden from our conscious mind may be numerous painful incidents where we have suppressed anger and frustration. Until these areas are recalled and specifically dealt with, God's healing process in our lives can be thwarted.

Certainly I could think of countless occasions when I had been hurt by others.

'But as far as I know I have forgiven everyone everything,' I said to Kenn. 'I don't think I'm harbouring any grudges.'

Kenn explained the importance of thinking of one person at a time, writing down every occasion when I had been hurt

by that person. Then I should go through that list one by one,
specifically forgiving the individual concerned for each hurt
caused, asking God to do the same, praying that God would
forgive me for my wrong reactions to those situations, calling
on the love of the Spirit to heal those wounds, and finally
inviting God to bless the person who hurt me. In this way I
could remove any blockages that were still there to God's
healing power.

'With some people I can think of, this is going to take ages!'
I said.

Kenn led me in prayer as I tried to deal with the hurts in
the past from one person, and then left me to continue the
process.

It is not always wise to investigate the causes of an illness,
but sometimes it may help. Canon Jim Glennon, who has
held powerful healing services in St Andrew's Cathedral,
Sydney for twenty-three years, wrote in a letter to me: 'Not
infrequently physical problems have emotional causes that
are linked to an event or events anything from six months to
two years before the onset of the physical consequence.'
Many doctors engaged in cancer research are of the same
opinion. Dr Carl Simonton, Director of Cancer Counselling
and Research Centre in Fort Worth writes: 'We believe that
cancer is often an indication of problems elsewhere in an
individual's life – problems aggravated and compounded by
a series of stresses, six to eighteen months prior to the onset of
cancer. The cancer patient has typically responded to these
problems and stresses with a deep sense of hopelessness or
"giving-up". This emotional response, we believe, in turn
triggers a set of physiological responses that suppress the
body's natural defences and make it susceptible to producing
abnormal cells.'[1] This may not be the only cause of cancer
but it is certainly worthy of serious consideration.

I thought back to one or two incidents in the past few years

[1]Quoted by Jim Glennon in *How Can I Find Healing?*, Hodder and
Stoughton, 1984.

that had wounded me very deeply, as well as many other conflicts and hurts in the past. It is impossible to say what the root cause of the cancer might be, but at least those hurts might have contributed to the breakdown of the immunity system. Another Christian friend remarked in a letter, 'One night as we were praying for you . . . I had the oddest feeling that you were suffering from a deep wound caused by the strife of tongues.' I immediately underlined that sentence when I read it. Certainly this is no time for recriminations, since these may only increase internal tensions and so aggravate the disease. When I am angry, in most cases I do not harm the person who has hurt me, but I rob myself of peace – and peace is integral to all healing.

Kenneth McCall once said that '*Fore-give-ness* is love given *before* another has either given it, earned it, accepted it, or even understood it.'[2] That is the nature of God's love, who sent his Son to bear our sins long before we ever thought of loving him. Love takes the initiative. When we have been hurt badly, we may not have the capacity to love the person who has distressed us. But God's love, which knows no such limitations, can be continuously poured into our hearts by the Holy Spirit.

I have described the inner healing that Kenn taught me only briefly, and if possible it is important to pray with a wise Christian counsellor who understands this process and has some experience. Although there could be a danger of introspection, it is much more like trying to get a splinter out of a finger. We have to probe a little, painful though it may be, until the foreign matter is removed. Bitterness is entirely foreign to God's purpose of wholeness for our lives. In the context of healing, the writer to Hebrews says 'Strive for peace with all men . . . that no "root of bitterness" spring up and cause trouble . . .' (12:14f). Unless we are willing to deal with any remaining bitterness in our hearts, we cannot rightly expect God to bring his healing and peace.

[2]*Healing the Family Tree.*

Someone wrote to me about a time when she had become aware of an unforgiving spirit in her heart. She repented of this, and asked for God's forgiveness and healing. 'But it was not until I got home that I realised that I was able to make movements easily and painlessly, that I had hitherto been either unable to make at all or had done so with pain!' She had been completely healed from arthritis in her lower back, and this came as soon as she had found peace in terms of her personal relationships.

I am still working through this area of inner healing, and I know that the sheer busyness of the last two months has so far prevented me from finishing the healing process that Kenn began. However I see the value of removing every hindrance to the work of God's Spirit in my life.

Recently I have had the most severe attack of asthma that I have known for many years. No medication seems to have affected it. Every night I wake up after about two hours of sleep, scarcely able to breathe. What is going on now? Is the cancer spreading to my lungs? Is it the result of a year of obvious stress, coupled with too many speaking engagements? I don't know.

Two nights ago, since I could not lie down to attempt to sleep, I prayed about every painful event and negative reaction from the past that I could think of (at least I made a start: two hours was far from sufficient). I confessed to God the times when I had both hurt and been hurt. I confessed that my rush back into normal work had begun to squeeze out my prayer routine. I confessed one or two relationships in which I still found it difficult to find peace. There was much more besides. It was a good time – like having a spiritual bath! Then I went to sleep, but woke breathless two hours later. This time I surrendered my life again to him, and listened to a worship cassette until I eventually fell back to sleep.

Why it all happened, I don't know. I record it simply as an indication that the battles do not seem to be over.

What is important – and what I gained from that rather

sleepless night – is that when we walk in love, our hearts, minds and bodies can be renewed daily by the Holy Spirit of love. The sooner we experience the healing of our emotions and relationships, the better we shall be able to attack the physical disease within us. At the very least we shall be at peace.

21

The Present Moment

Eleven months have passed since the cancer in my body was first detected – eleven months of the limited life I am expected to have left, the original sentence being about one year. The medical prognosis is still the same, and the latest scan showed a further increase in the tumour. The future officially is bleak, and I am getting used to people looking at me as a dying man under sentence of death. Nothing is certain. I'm not out of the wood yet. Everything is a matter of faith.

That is why I have written the book at this stage. I am not looking back at a painful episode in the past; the difficulties are still with me. I am not writing from a position of comparative safety; I am at present in the thick of it, with humanly speaking no answers, no certainties, no proof of healing – nothing except a somewhat daunting unknown. And yet in reality, my position is not fundamentally different from that of anyone else. No one knows what the future holds. Our lives are full of ifs and buts and supposings. Nothing is sure apart from death. Whether we like it or not, everyone has to live by faith. The *object* of faith is naturally of absolute importance, and may vary considerably. Some will trust in God, others in money, luck, prosperity, health, medicine, philosophy or wishful thinking. But no one can escape the risk of faith when it comes to the greatest issues of life and death.

The opposite to faith is fear, and I have found that there is a constant running battle between the two. In one sense, fear is faith in what you do not want to happen. Job once said, 'The thing I fear comes upon me, and what I dread befalls me' (3:25). There is a powerful truth in that statement. When we are afraid of something, we almost pre-condition it to happen. Our fears, however unfounded and irrational they may be, can trigger the fulfilment of those fears.

Fear has been described as the greatest threat to health in our generation, simply because fear is so widespread. Fear is a great deceiver and destroyer. It robs our minds of peace; it distorts our understanding; it magnifies our problems; it breaks our relationships; it ruins our health; it goads us into foolish, impulsive and sometimes violent action; it paralyses our thinking, trusting and loving.

Repeatedly Jesus had to rebuke his disciples for their fears and lack of faith: 'Why are you afraid? Have you no faith?' (Mark 4:40). The context of that particular challenge is interesting. The disciples were in a boat, caught in a violent storm on the Sea of Galilee; and even though some of them were tough and experienced fishermen, they were scared stiff. So they woke Jesus, who was asleep in the boat: 'Teacher, do you not care if we perish?' It seemed to them that he did not care, since he was sleeping peacefully in the tempest. At once Jesus rebuked the wind and the waves, and there was a great calm. But Jesus was clearly disappointed that his disciples had not yet learned to trust God in the midst of their difficulties. '*Why* are you afraid?'

God never promises to protect us from problems, only to help us in them. If we leave God out of the picture, those difficulties might so strip away our sense of security that we feel vulnerable, anxious and afraid. On the other hand, those same difficulties could drive us back to God and so strengthen our faith. We might feel just as vulnerable, but we *have* to trust God because there is really no alternative; and then we discover that God is with us in the dark as in the light, in pain as in joy. When I was going through a traumatic time in my life, a friend of mine said, 'You cannot trust God too much.'

What we may not realise is how much we are trapped by

our own thoughts and words. If we fill our minds with
negative ideas, we may plunge into self-pity, despondency or
fear. Even our bodies may react negatively with disease. The
more we reflect on our hurts, the more we shall be bound by
bitterness and prone to physical afflictions, such as arthritis.
If we fail in some task and dwell upon that failure, we may get
angry with ourselves (and no doubt angry with others also),
and this could precipitate deep depression – depression is
often a matter of suppressed anger. The more we think about
our fears, or express them to others, the more gripped by
anxiety we shall become, to the point of crippling phobias.

I have had to watch all this carefully over the last eleven
months. When I've had a difficult day or week, I sometimes
find myself saying, especially in the middle of the night, 'I've
got cancer, it's spreading and I'm dying. How am I going to
tell the children?' At times like these I sweat a bit. But when I
am more awake I realise that negative thoughts only accelerate the disease and could lead to an early death. How then
should I control my thoughts? Should I say instead, 'I'm fit
and well and there's nothing wrong with me at all?' That
would be a positive remark and possibly beneficial; but it is
not an honest statement and has no substance apart from
wishful thinking. It might be called 'faith', but it's a dangerous faith without any solid foundation. That is the weakness
of those who teach 'the power of positive thinking'. Without
any doubt positive thinking is far better than negative, but
the question remains: what are the grounds for such definite
thoughts? What is the basis of such faith?

As a Christian I am called to rest my faith firmly on God
and on the promises of God's word. Jesus said that this was
the solid rock on which the house of my life would stand firm
against even the fiercest storms. Constantly Jesus endorsed
the authority of God's word: he knew it, taught it, lived by it,
and corrected his opponents by bringing them back to the
truth of it: 'You are wrong, because you know neither the
scriptures nor the power of God' (Matthew 22:29). Here too
was the basis of faith for the apostles and the early Church:

they knew that God was faithful and that his word could not be broken. Convinced of the ultimate reality of this, they went through fire and water, torture and martyrdom, because they knew that nothing at all could ever separate them from the love of God in Christ Jesus (see Romans 8:28–39 and Hebrews 11).

This has also been the faith that has sustained countless Christians down the centuries, many of whom have suffered acutely for their commitment to Christ. Martin Niemöller was incarcerated in a Nazi concentration camp for many years, but was allowed the Bible as his one possession. He wrote: 'The Bible: what did this book mean to me during the long and weary years of solitary confinement and then for the last four years at Dachau cell-building? The word of God was simply everything to me – comfort and strength, guidance and hope, master of my days and companion of my nights, the bread which kept me from starvation, and the water of life which refreshed my soul. And even more, "solitary confinement" ceased to be solitary.' This is the constant experience of those who have dared to take God at his word, despite all the odds against them.

In order to maintain a positive faith and not give way to negative fears, I have found it important to go on thanking God for the truth of his word and for the power of his Spirit at work within me. When I am asked (as I often am), 'How are you?' I reply truthfully, 'I'm feeling fine, and I believe that God is continuing to heal me. But I should be grateful for your prayers.' That is where my faith stands. From God's word I do not doubt that he wants to heal me, and there have also been personal assurances of this healing through the remarks of many Christians from all over the world. Of course I realise that logically speaking we may all be wrong. But my faith is neither groundless nor mindless. I have good reason for believing that God *is* healing me, and I shall go on trusting him and praising him whatever I may be feeling like. I cannot honestly say 'I *have* been healed' because there is no medical evidence to support that at present. A few Christians have written (rather unhelpfully) rebuking me for my lack of faith in not accepting that healing is now an accomplished fact. However, I can only be honest with where I am; and since my faith is in a God who is not limited by the scientific world-view I believe that God *is* healing me, and I am accepting many engagements for the next year or two without thinking too much about the 'risk' entailed. From a Christian perspective, that seems to be both a reasonable and a responsible position of faith.

Nevertheless, I am aware of the spiritual battle involved. I was temporarily thrown when a close Christian friend of mine asked if I was booking a reserve speaker for my various engagements. I knew he was deeply concerned to remove all extra pressures from me, but his question still disturbed me. There is admittedly a fine dividing line between faith and foolishness, but how could I genuinely believe in God's healing if I were at the same time booking an alternative speaker in case I were ill?

At the end of September I went with my team to the beautiful Bernese Oberland in Switzerland to lead a week's conference for Christian pastors and workers. It proved a wonderful week. In spite of everything having to be translated into German (which none of our team spoke), the sense of God's presence and the joy of Christian fellowship was almost breathtaking. There were pastors from Eastern Germany and Poland too, which added to the quality of the week. As a special bonus we had an afternoon cruising down Lake Thun, a day in Bern (surely the most beautiful capital in the world), and another day up the mountains overlooking the Eiger and Jungfrau. Ironically, all previous English speakers invited to this annual conference had cancelled, sometimes at the last moment. I was the only one who actually made it, even though no one was entirely certain about this until we arrived! I am glad to say that no alternative speaker had been booked on this occasion!

In October I found myself speaking at a number of special lunches, dinners, services and festivals where there were

excellent numbers and an unusual degree of interest, no
doubt partly due to my illness. My autobiography *You Are My
God*, published on October 3rd, had record sales, running
into its fifth printing by the end of that month! Also I had
more interviews on radio and for the press than I had known
during several years put together. I thought again of that
prophetic word given before my operation that my future
ministry would increase rather than decrease.

'What if you are not healed?' I am sometimes asked.
Although it does not help to dwell on that question too much,
I realise that it is a perfectly fair one; and that is where the
Christian hope for the future is so enormously important. Of
course I cannot *know* that I shall have ten to twenty years
more to live. I cannot *know* that I have even one. But that is
also true of every one of us. With all our planning for the
future, we need to live a day at a time and enjoy each day as a
gift from God. 'This is the day which the Lord has made; let
us rejoice and be glad in it' (Psalm 118:24). Some Christians
speak of the *sacrament of the present moment*: we need to live, not
just a day at a time, but moment by moment, seeking to do
God's will for each moment of our life. That alone is the way
in which we can know the fullness of God's joy and peace.

'What about those who are praying for you, if you are not
healed? Will not their faith be severely shaken, if they are so
convinced that you will be well?' Once again, that is a
reasonable question. My answer is that it's God's responsibility! God is so much bigger than our mistakes. Indeed our
relationship with him deepens only when we work through
disappointments, confusion, bewilderment and, at times,
despair. I cannot let the thought of 'disappointing those who
are praying for me' become a negative pressure in my life. I
am delighted that so many *are* praying for me, and I believe
that their prayers are being answered. If I am wrong, God is
well able to handle that one. He has had plenty of experience!

In the Bible, one shining example of faith is Abraham who
left his homeland in obedience to God, and who trusted
God's promise of a son even when he was 100 years old and

his wife ninety. The apostle Paul made this comment about Abraham: 'No distrust made him waver concerning the promise of God, but he grew strong in his faith as he gave glory to God, fully convinced that God was able to do what he had promised' (Romans 4:20f). The tense of the Greek verb suggests that as Abraham *went on* giving glory to God (i.e. praising God), his faith became strong and the miracle happened.

This is the way in which we encourage our faith. Basing our trust on the assurance of God's word and faithfulness, we continue to praise God for the truth of his word until it is fulfilled. In Hebrews 11, the great chapter on faith, the writer acknowledges that sometimes faith is not rewarded this side of heaven. But whatever the size of the problem, the length of the battle, or the outcome of our faith, we are called to trust in God and to keep our eyes on Jesus.

That, after all, is the ultimate purpose of our life. 'Eternal life', said Jesus when praying, 'means knowing you, the only true God, and knowing Jesus Christ whom you sent' (John 17:3, *Good News Bible*). Nothing is more important than our relationship with God, both for this life and for the next.

A doctor complained recently, 'Our patients expect us to make them immortal!' Many cling tenaciously to this life because they fear there is nothing more to come. Today's preoccupation with youth and youthfulness demonstrates the same deep-seated anxiety about the future, especially that last enemy death, of which cancer seems the most frightening symbol.

One day we stand to lose everything of this world, and no one knows when that day will come. Once we have lost our lives to God, however, we belong eternally to him; and in Christ we have all that is ultimately important. If we spend our time worrying about ourselves, we have missed the whole point of our existence. C. S. Lewis expressed it like this: 'Look for yourself, and in that long run you will find only hatred, loneliness, despair, rage, ruin and decay. But look for Christ and you will find him, and with him everything else thrown in.'[1] That is the only security that ultimately makes sense.

God offers no promise to shield us from the evil of this fallen world. There is no immunity guaranteed from sickness, pain, sorrow or death. What he does pledge is his never-failing presence for those who have found him in Christ. Nothing can destroy that. Always he is with us. And, in the long run, that is all we need to know.

[1] *Mere Christianity*, Fountain Books, 1952.

22

What Happens at Death?

Faced with terminal cancer and with the medical prognosis of an early death, I thought carefully about the perpetually puzzling question, what happens at death? When the moment comes – as it will for every one of us sooner or later, whether we think about it or not – what will be the experience of death and what, if anything, lies beyond it?

Philosophers, writers and poets down the centuries have always been intrigued by this question. Job asked, 'If a man dies shall he live again?' John Betjeman, in one of his poems imagines himself waiting for an operation, and wonders, 'is it extinction when I die?'

Some state dogmatically that extinction is all that we can expect. Bertrand Russell talked about the 'night of nothingness': 'There is darkness without and when I die there will be darkness within. There is no splendour, no vastness, anywhere; only triviality for a moment, and then nothing.'[1]

All this, of course, is pure theory. By our own wisdom we do not *know* what happens at death. We cannot, since it lies beyond our present experience and outside the limits of human knowledge. Indeed, the mystery surrounding death has no doubt been partly responsible for such a growing interest in spiritualism and in occult practices in general. In the absence of a living Christian hope, the vacuum has to be filled with some alternative, however unsatisfactory. After the death of my father I dabbled in a few séances myself, to

[1] *Autobiography*, vol. 2, George Allen and Unwin, London, 1968.

see if I could get in touch with him. I have since become
aware of the considerable dangers of such practices, and the
Bible gives wise and clear warnings about them.

The cruel and inescapable fact of death, however, causes
many people to consider carefully the meaning of their lives.
When I was in New Zealand in 1973 I read this fascinating
comment in a newspaper article by the Director of radio-
therapy and radiology in that country:

> Cancer makes people start thinking about the quality of
> their lives. Everything they do has a keener edge on it and
> they get more out of life. In fact some people never become
> completely human beings and really start living until they
> get cancer. We all know we are going to die some time, but
> cancer makes people face up to it . . . They are going to go
> on living with a lot of extra enjoyment, just because they
> have faced the fear of death. Cancer patients aren't dying.
> They're living. I h ve never seen a suicide because of
> cancer.[2]

That has certainly been my own experience, and I am much
more aware of the value of each day, and the importance of
making good use of it. The quality of my life has far from
diminished. Philosophers have always maintained that the
key to life is coming to terms with death. No one can live well
until they can die well. In the famous words of Samuel
Johnson, 'When a man knows he is to be hanged in a
fortnight, it concentrates his mind wonderfully!' Certainly all
the great issues of life and death come into sharp focus when
the future is known to be precarious.

What is the nature of death? There is much confusion
about this, understandably, and the Bible significantly talks
about 'the shadow of death'. We do not see clearly what it is,
nor what lies ahead of us. Sometimes death is referred to as a
horizon. A horizon marks the limit of what I can see now, but

[2]Quoted in the *Palmerston North Evening Standard*, June 7th, 1973.

does not mark the limit of where I can go later. There is something beyond a horizon.

The essence of death is *separation*, and the Bible distinguishes three forms of death.

First there is *spiritual death*, when we find ourselves, naturally through our sin, separated from God. If I go my way and not God's, it stands to reason that I shall separate myself from him. That is why God often seems so remote and so unreal. God's answer to spiritual death, as we have already seen in this book, is the offer of spiritual life through the cross of Jesus Christ. Christ died to bring us to God, so that we might know God and enjoy his love for ever. Nothing can ever separate us from that love, once we have come to him through Jesus Christ.

Secondly, there is *physical death*, when the soul is separated from the body, and the person is separated from family and friends. When two people get married it is 'till death us do part'. Death ruthlessly breaks the deepest bonds of love. God's answer to physical death is that, instead of a physical body which is subject to pain and sickness, weariness and decay, he gives us a spiritual or resurrection body. In Paul's great chapter on this theme (1 Corinthians 15), he takes the analogy of a seed sown in the ground and dying before it can bear fruit, and he writes: 'What is sown is perishable, what is raised is imperishable. It is sown in dishonour, it is raised in glory. It is sown in weakness, it is raised in power. It is sown a physical body, it is raised a spiritual body.' There is scarcely any resemblance between a small seed sown in the ground and the lovely flower developing from it. Had we no previous experience, it would be impossible to imagine the transformed beauty of the flower by looking carefully at the small and unimpressive seed. Yet there is a continuity between the two. Out of death springs a much more glorious life. So it is with our spiritual body.

It is obviously impossible to describe precisely what this resurrection body will be like, since we do not yet have any first-hand experience of it. Perhaps our nearest hint is the resurrection body of Jesus which was clearly recognisable to his friends, and yet different. He could pass through locked doors; he could both appear and vanish at will. Professor Donald Mackay of Keele University, one of Britain's foremost experts on the communication system of the human brain, has made this interesting comment:

> It is not as disembodied spirits that God promises us eternal life, but as personalities expressed in a new kind of body – what the apostle Paul calls a 'spiritual body'. Just as a message is still the same message, whether it is spoken in words or flashed in morse code, so, according to the Bible, we shall be the same persons, whatever the material form in which our personalities may be expressed. Nothing in the scientific picture of man, however complete it may one day become, could affect the truth of this doctrine one way or another.[3]

Thirdly, there is *eternal death*, which means total separation from God and from all good. When the sun shines with strength, the plants with their roots in the soil grow and flourish, but the plants without their roots in the soil wither and die. It is a natural law; it is also a spiritual law. If we are not rooted and grounded in the love of God, we cannot escape his righteous judgment. The essence of God's judgment is that, with infinite sadness, he underlines the decision that *we* make about him. If we rule God out of our lives, we are ruled out of his life. That is our decision, not his. In his great love for us, he has sent his only Son so that we might never have to face the appalling consequences of his judgment; but if we do not want his forgiveness, we shall not have it. If I do not want God in my life I will not know him.

However, God's answer to eternal death is the free offer of eternal life through Jesus Christ, based on the solid assurance of Christ's resurrection. The apostle Peter put it like

[3]From an essay in *Inter-Varsity*, 1970.

this: 'Blessed be the God and Father of our Lord Jesus Christ! By his great mercy we have been born anew to a living hope through the resurrection of Jesus Christ from the dead, and to an inheritance which is imperishable, undefiled, and unfading, kept in heaven for you' (1 Peter 1:3f). Paul too had a longing to depart this life and to be with Christ, which he knew would be 'far better' than anything that he could experience on this earth.

For those who have put their trust in Christ now, death means that we shall be perfectly with him, more alive than ever, and free from pain, sickness, anxiety, depression and sin. On the memorial of Martin Luther King are these simple words:

Rev Martin Luther King Jr
1929–1968
'Free at last, free at last,
Thank God A'mighty I'm free at last'

The Church is the only society on earth that never loses a member through death! As a Christian I believe, not just in life *after* death, but in life *through* death. In the words of a Russian Christian, 'The moment of death will be the inrush of timelessness.'

What happens at death? It is of course impossible to answer this with any precision, since we cannot draw from past experience. The Bible speaks in general terms, necessarily using metaphors and pictures, although the underlying truth of these is clear.

From the teaching of Jesus, it seems that at the moment of death there will be a *great divide* between those who know and love God, and those who do not. An amazing number of parables alone indicate this division: the wheat and the tares, the sheep and the goats, the great banquet, the rich fool, the wise and foolish bridesmaids, those with or without wedding garments, the drag net of good and bad fish, the house on the rock and the house on the sand. 'The message of Jesus is not only the proclamation of salvation, but the announcement of judgment, a cry of warning and a call to repentance in view of the terrible urgency of the crisis. The number of parables in this category is nothing less than awe-inspiring.'[4] It is impossible to escape this basic truth which rings repeatedly throughout the Gospel records.

In one of his most telling parables (Luke 16:19–31) Jesus spoke of two men who died. One was comfortably rich, deaf to God and blind to the needy; the other was wretchedly poor, trusting only in the mercy of God. At death a great chasm was fixed between them, the rich man in hell and the poor man in heaven. It was impossible to cross from one side to the other – there is no suggestion anywhere in the Bible of a second chance after death. The rich man in torment becomes concerned about the spiritual state of his five brothers. He was told that they, like all of us, had the clear warnings of scripture. If we ignore these, nothing will persuade us, not even someone returning from the dead. With all the metaphorical language taken into account, the teaching about God's judgment after death is so unmistakably clear, especially in the teaching of Jesus, that we have only ourselves to blame if we ignore it.

C. S. Lewis once saw this epitaph on a tombstone:

> Here lies an atheist
> all dressed up but
> with nowhere to go.

Lewis added his own comment, 'I bet he wishes that were so.'

It is important to add, however, that Jesus also indicated that God's judgment depends on the opportunity we have had to respond to his love and mercy (Luke 12:47f). Since God has revealed himself in some measure to everyone in this world, at least through creation and conscience (see Romans 1:18–32 and 2:1–16), no one is without excuse. However,

[4] J. Jeremias.

without attempting to be dogmatic, it is my personal belief that those who put their trust in God's love and mercy *insofar as they understand him*, will be accepted by him. As a motorist may cross a bridge on a motorway without realising that the bridge is even there (let alone any details about it), so it may be possible for a person to come to God 'over the bridge' of Christ without knowing anything about him. That person's understanding, joy, assurance, faith and hope will all naturally be limited, until he does discover the truth about Christ. But personally I do not believe from the scriptures that there is no hope at all for those who do not, or cannot, call themselves Christians. If in their hearts they have truly responded to God, however little they know about his Son or his gift of salvation, God may well accept them on that Day of Judgment. What *is* clear, however, is that those of us who do know, or can know, have no excuse whatsoever if we 'neglect so great a salvation' (Hebrews 2:3). At least we can rest assured that God, who is Judge over all the earth, will do what is right.

Certainly, for those who die in Christ the future will be unimaginably wonderful. The expression used several times is 'falling asleep' (see 1 Thessalonians 4:13–18; 1 Corinthians 15:20). When we fall asleep after a tiring day, the next thing we know is waking refreshed the following morning. So it will be for the Christian. We fall asleep in Christ, and then wake up on the resurrection morning with our new spiritual bodies.

From a human perspective, hundreds of years may have elapsed between death and resurrection. But time is a human limitation. God is essentially outside time. 'With the Lord one day is as a thousand years, and a thousand years as one day' (2 Peter 3:8). When Jesus was hanging on the cross, he promised the dying thief who cried to him for help, 'Truly, I say to you, *today* you will be with me in Paradise' (Luke 23:43). Time is relative to motion, as Einstein has shown us. For example, at the speed of light the passage of time vanishes. Everything happens now! Subject as we are to the dimensions of time during this life, the concept of a timeless eternity is hard, if not impossible, to grasp. We can therefore only grope for metaphors and pictures about heaven.

We cannot know exactly what we shall be like after death. The apostle John put it like this: 'It is not yet clear what we shall become. But we know that when Christ appears, we shall be like him, because we shall see him as he really is' (1 John 3:2, *Good News Bible*). That should be sufficient for us. Heaven is being 'with Christ' when we shall be 'like him'. There will be a wonderful sense of being fully in God's presence, in an unspoilt and unbroken atmosphere of love, joy and praise.

If we think of all the best and most glorious moments in our lives, the perfection of what we experience always seems just beyond our reach. As with striking a succession of matches to light a dark room, those moments invariably seem to flicker and fade. Heaven will be like turning on the full light. The perfection will be there for us to enjoy, undefiled, unflickering and unfading. 'And the city had no need of sun or moon to shine upon it, for the glory of God is its light . . .' (Revelation 21:23). Here is the summit of all our highest hopes and dreams.

In one sense, the Christian is not preparing for death. Essentially he is preparing for *life*, abundant life in all its fullness. The world, with its fleeting pleasures, is not the final reality, with heaven as a shadowy and suspect unknown. The best and purest joys on earth are only a shadow of the reality that God has prepared for us in Christ. Eternal life begins as soon as we receive Christ as our Saviour. We can start enjoying it now, in increasing measure, and should be preparing, not for death, but for the consummation of that perfect quality of life when we are completely in God's presence for ever. Quantity of life is not nearly so important as quality, even for 'terminally ill' patients. By the way, I don't like that word 'terminal', which means the end of something. In reality, when the body of the Christian dies, the really wonderful journey has only just begun. Even my secular dictionary defines heaven as 'a place or state of supreme bliss.' So it is.

Death for the Christian, it is sometimes said, is like the old family servant who opens the door to welcome the children home. Although it would be a mistake to base our beliefs on the experience of those who have clinically died but later have been restored to life, it is worth noting that of those who were Christians nearly all speak of walking peacefully into a garden full of staggeringly beautiful colours and exquisite music (or some similar description), so that it was with great reluctance that they came back to earth again.

It never worries me that we are not able to grasp more clearly the true nature of heaven. We can understand something of which we have no first-hand experience only by describing something with which we are familiar. We are limited by language. But for those who know God and who are trusting in Christ as their Saviour and Lord, there is nothing to fear, and it is sufficient to know that we shall be like him and perfectly with him. Nothing could be more wonderful than that. Never fear the worst. *The best is yet to be.*

When I die, it is my firm conviction that I shall be more alive than ever, experiencing the full reality of all that God has prepared for us in Christ. Sometimes I have foretastes of that reality, when the sense of God's presence is especially vivid. Although such moments are comparatively rare they whet my appetite for much more. The actual moment of dying is still shrouded in mystery, but as I keep my eyes on Jesus I am not afraid. Jesus has already been through death for us, and will be with us when we walk through it ourselves. In those great words of the Twenty-Third Psalm:

> Even though I walk through the valley
>   of the shadow of death,
>   I fear no evil;
>   for thou art with me . . .

January 1984

Any struggle with cancer and death is likely to have unexpected twists and turns. A sudden burst of joy when dark clouds that threaten a raging storm give way to sunshine and springtime hopefulness. Or just the reverse when our faith and hope are plunged into that ugly pit of depression.

When I sent the manuscript of this book to the publishers I was feeling remarkably fit, apart from the puzzling backache that had bothered me for three or four months. 'How well you look!' everyone said to me. And I felt it. My waist was trim, my appetite good – I felt thoroughly *alive*!

Abruptly everything changed.

With the enjoyment of being back at work again, especially with my team, I threw my new energies into all that I could. After the Pastors' Conference in Switzerland, we had exciting visits to Manchester, the Isle of Wight, Belfast and Dublin, plenty of preaching engagements in London, as well as some broadcasting and writing. I knew it was too much, but everywhere we went the crowds and enthusiasm exceeded all expectations. At a Diocesan Service of Renewal in Southwark Cathedral (which seats 800) an estimated crowd of 2000 turned up. Autumn '83 was a time when God seemed to be working with unusual power.

Then my body protested against all this activity by the most severe attack of asthma I have had for many years. In the past, such attacks had been controlled quickly by a certain course of steroids. I took this again, but my asthma continued unchecked, giving me broken nights and much discomfort. One side-effect was a thoroughly unpleasant development of thrush in my mouth during our Irish tour.

Still my asthma got worse. So I was given the highest dose
of steroids I have ever had, which again aggravated the
thrush. So with the generosity of some close friends and with
the encouragement of many (including Anne) I flew over to
California for special prayer at John Wimber's church, since
I felt I was losing the battle.

I was there for only eight days, and they were marvellous
in their love, concern and prayer support. Each day different
teams of Christians, experienced in the healing ministry,
prayed for me, for periods ranging from two to five hours a
day. Yet, for whatever reason, everything seemed to get
worse. The asthma persisted, so that I slept badly each night;
my legs, ankles and feet blew up like balloons; and my
abdomen grew at an astonishing rate until I looked like a
pregnant woman in about her seventh month! My arms and
shoulders withered into mere skin and bones, and instead of
returning from California bursting with new health (as I had
expected), I looked more dead than alive.

Drastic changes had to be made. Virtually all speaking
engagements for the future were cancelled immediately,
including major events in California, Norway, Sweden and
Vancouver – which had been carefully planned for anything
up to two years previously. My team would have to be
disbanded by the end of April at the latest. I was now literally
fighting for my life.

'God hasn't done anything for David,' people are now
beginning to say. 'We've prayed and prayed, and nothing
has happened at all.' Medically speaking, that seems to be
true. I am a fairly typical cancer patient with secondaries in
the liver. Temporary remissions may occur, but then everything may suddenly 'explode'. At the moment there is still
some uncertainty as to which symptoms are due to the
steroids, having been on these for almost two months (I took
my last one, I hope, this morning and the asthma is better).
But there is no doubt that my liver has considerably enlarged
due to sudden activity of the cancer cells.

However God has been far from inactive in my life. At

about one a.m. on Advent Sunday morning, I had a bad
asthmatic attack. In my helplessness, I cried out to God to
speak to me. I'm not very good at listening to God, but
between one and three a.m. God spoke to me so powerfully
and painfully that I have never felt so broken before him (and
still do).

He showed me that all my preaching, writing and other
ministry was absolutely *nothing* compared to my love-
relationship with him. In fact, my sheer busyness had
squeezed out the close intimacy I had known with him
during the first few months of the year after my operation.

God also showed me that any 'love' for him meant *nothing*
unless I was truly able to love from my heart my brother or
sister in Christ. As the Lord put various names into my mind
I began to write letters to about twelve people asking for
forgiveness for hurting them, for still being inwardly angry
against them – or whatever. It was the most painful pruning
and purging I can remember in my entire Christian life. But
fruitful! Already some replies to my letters have reduced me
to tears.

Whatever else is happening to me physically, God is
working deeply in my life. His challenge to me can be
summed up in three words: 'Seek my face.' I am not now
clinging to physical life (though I still believe that God can
heal and wants to heal); but I am clinging to the Lord. I am
ready to go and to be with Christ for ever. That would be
literally heaven. But I'm equally ready to stay, if that is what
God wants.

'Father, not my will but yours be done.' In that position of
security I have experienced once again his perfect love, a love
that casts out all fear.

Epilogue

David wrote the last pages of this book during the first week of January 1984.

On January 8th he preached at St Michael's, Chester Square, from Jude verses 20–5. He said:

> The last couple of months have seen some pretty sweeping changes in my own life. I have had to cancel all my engagements outside London and after travelling for many years I would have found that very difficult if it had not been for God so clearly calling me back to this love relationship with him. Even death itself is not a threat.

On January 15th he preached again at St Michael's, this time on Psalm 91, which he found 'highy relevant'.

> He who dwells in the shelter of the Most High,
>> Who abides in the shadow of the Almighty,
> Will say to the Lord, 'My refuge and my fortress;
>> My God in whom I trust.'

From January 16th David's condition deteriorated rapidly. He continued to see close friends from time to time and on Monday 30th he said to David MacInnes: 'I am completely at peace – there is nothing that I want more than to go to heaven. I know how good it is.'

David remained at home nursed by Anne and her mother. He saw members of his team when they returned from five weeks in California, and especially enjoyed times with his children. Late on the evening of Friday, 17th February he said to Anne: 'I'm very tired; let's go home.'

*   *   *

David Watson died peacefully very early next morning, February 18th.

'The Lord Reigns'